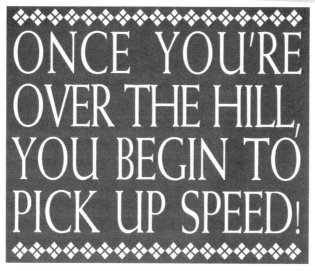

ONCE YOU'RE OVER THE HILL, YOU BEGIN TO PICK UP SPEED!

Selma Jacob

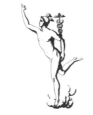

HEALTH PRESS
PO BOX 1388
SANTA FE, NEW MEXICO 87504

Title used with permission from Charles M. Schulz

Published by Health Press
P.O. Drawer 1388
Santa Fe, NM 87504

96 95 94 93 92   5 4 3 2 1

ii

❖

Library of Congress Cataloging-in-Publication Data

Jacob, Selma, 1905
Once You're Over the Hill, You Begin To Pick Up Speed!
        Selma Jacob
                p.   cm.

        ISBN 0-929173-12-0

                1. Humor. 2. Elder Issues.
I. Title.
                [   ]

Cover and book design by Suzanne Vilmain
Edited by Denice Anderson
Opinions stated herein are those of the author
and do not necessarily reflect the position of Health Press.

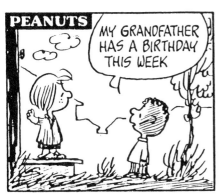
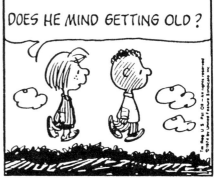
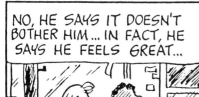
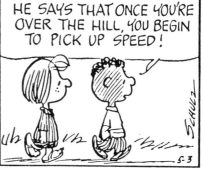
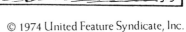

iii

❖

ACKNOWLEDGEMENTS

They say that, consciously or unconsciously, we pick up something from everyone with whom we come in contact.

I have been so fortunate to have come in contact with the following people from whom I learned so much, or who encouraged me to do things!

Lorraine Allen, the epitome of sophistication and a great commercial designer and artist for General Electric. Marge and Bob Kohn, my attorney, whose repeated encouragement almost amounted to nagging - and Ona and David Owen, for the same reason. My cousin, Elise Newman, whose knowledge of all forms of art is exceeded by none. Gary Tipton, who together with Actors' Theatre of Louisville, and Georgette Kleier, David Palmer, Bertram Harris of the University of Louisville's Department of Dramatic Arts taught me so much about theatre, and what a wonderful world it is - Paul Owen, set designer extraordinaire and great artist, at Actors' Theatre of Louisville; Ken Pyle and Sheila Joyce of The Rudyard Kipling Dinner Theatre. The Louisville Writers, the Arts Club of Louisville, Dr. Leon Driskell, Charles Keefe, curator of Brown County Gallery, Indiana, were all fine teachers. The valets, security guards, maintenance crew and personnel at 1400 Willow and Ray Broad and Sheila Rockey who are a constant source of joy and helpfulness. The two most helpful and most beloved groups of all, my own "Writers and Readers" and "Drama Study Group," composed of two great assemblies of helpful delightful people: I love each one. I give my sincerest thanks and gratitude to these people without whom this book would still be a pile of blank paper.

And a great big "Thank You" to Charles M. Schulz for permission to use his quote and cartoon, "Once You're Over The Hill, You Begin To Pick Up Speed!" which is so true.

PREFACE

If you were to look up "Selma Jacob" in the dictionary (where she wouldn't be) you would find (which you won't) that I am an eighty-seven-year-old woman who spent my life just outside the perimeter of all the things I loved, such as painting, writing, and the theater. Until I retired in 1984, I never had the opportunity to pursue these things because the 1929 stock market crash swallowed everything, leaving only the indigestible harshness of a struggle to stay alive.

Before the depression, I spent two informative years in New York when American theater, the Algonquin Round Table, the New Yorker Magazine with Harold Ross, the Roxy, Rockefeller Center, Schubert's Winter Garden, and all the most brilliant novelists, playwrights, actors, artists, and producers were at the height of their glory.

After the crash, I returned to Louisville, where, born and reared, I have continued to live.

One evening, at dinner with my attorney, Robert Kohn, I was was persuaded to write a book. He said, "You have a special attitude toward life. Pass it along!"

The book wrote itself rapidly, as there was no research to be done. The material all came from within me from my life, thoughts and experiences.

It has all been proven.

It works.

It will work for you.

Hope you enjoy it.

— Selma Jacob

v

❖

CONTENTS

vi

vii

BOOK TWO
Mellow Maturity Section
page 25

BOOK THREE
Memories Section
page 47

ix

❖

BOOK ONE *Philosophy*

I have a simple philosophy.
Fill what's empty. Empty what's full.
And scratch where it itches.

— Alice Roosevelt Longworth

And remember this:
You can't change the past
But you can ruin the present
By worrying about the future.

— Selma Jacob

1

1
You Don't Have To Act
To Be A Shakespearean

When I was very young, I went to Sunday school and heard, "Do unto others as you would have others do unto you," and I was terribly impressed. That was good stuff. I liked it. The Golden Rule. Everybody should obey it, and there wouldn't be any trouble. It seems a good rule to live by.

A bit later I heard, "This above all: to thine own self be true, and it must follow, as the night the day, thou canst not then be false to any man." I thought, "Oh my! That's great. That's as great as the Golden Rule." I was sure it was from the <u>Bible</u>. Where else could such wisdom—such excellent advice—come from?

I decided that this quotation and the Golden Rule were all I needed to live by. The route of my life was set. With these two guidelines to steer me, my destination was bound to be Nirvana, Camelot, or at least "The Good Ship Lollipop."

Later I learned that "This above all: to thine own self be true" was Polonius's speech in *Hamlet*. I was so surprised. I felt sure it was from the <u>Bible</u>. Then when people would say to me, "You seem to have your own definite ideas about life and religion. What are you? Jewish? Catholic? Presbyterian?" I'd say, "I'm Shakespearean!"

2
Uneasy Lies And The Head
That Lies – And Lies – And Lies

I married such a nice fellow. He had so many good qualities. When I met him, there were just a few things (relatively minor, but important to me) about him that I thought could be improved, and I knew it would be a simple thing to change them after we were married. There was a song from a musical that was very popular at the time: "Marry the man to-day. Change him around to-morrow." That seemed to be the theme song for most brides-to-be.

The trouble was, *I* had several qualities that could be improved upon; although, I didn't realize it. And do you know what happened? Before I had a chance to change him, *he* changed *me*. Now don't you think that was deceitful? How dishonest can you get?

"By and large" I was an honest person but "nearby and small" I was not above telling a wee falsehood, as a matter of convenience rather than as a matter of malice. If a little statement that wasn't quite the absolute truth served a purpose in a more satisfying way than having to be boldly honest, well, why not?

When these little social lies began to put me in a spot of embarrassment, Hy said to me, "Look. You're very foolish. You don't have to lie. You don't have to put yourself in an unpleasant spot. Tell the truth. Always be in the clear. You will feel much more secure. If there's any discomfort, it needn't be yours." How could I have forgotten "This above all: to thine own self be true"? This advice emphasized the strength of it.

For the past sixty-five years, I have never told even the tiniest white lie. It's a wonderful feeling. Priceless.

Please don't tell a lie. Not even a tiny one.

This may bring up the situation, "I told her the truth about herself, and she was offended. You mean to tell me I haven't the right to express my opinion? I have a right to say what I think, don't I?" The answer is, "No. You don't."

There is a great difference between being a truthful person and being a blabbermouth. A successful person considers carefully what positive, or at least noncommittal, remark can be made or tactfully introduces another subject.

If you want to be respected and beloved, do not lie–and do not be a blabbermouth.

Again, it is important to think before you speak. If the remark is better left unsaid, don't say it.

❖

3

You Are A Huge Fingerprint – There's No One Else In the World Exactly Like You

Sometimes it's difficult to live with other people, so aren't you lucky that there's no one under your skin but you. No one has control of your body but you. No one has your brain but you. You are the only one who can control your mind.

Isn't it wonderful that you always have a choice, and the choice can *always* be a positive one.

It's true that some people hate positive thoughts because they stand in the way of their being miserable. Don't be like that. If you're not going to have fun, who is going to have it for you?

Many people feel that a single man has an advantage over a single woman in that he can go places alone, such as to restaurants, to the theater, or on trips, but don't you believe it. If a woman confidently holds her head high and conducts herself with dignity, there isn't anyplace that a man can go where she can't go, except, perhaps, to a few bars or Turkish baths or all of the men's rest rooms.

"If you don't have a pleasant time and as much fun as you can— as long as it doesn't harm you or anyone else–you are cheating yourself and often those around you. That isn't fair." That was one of my husband Hy's and my grandparent's favorite sayings. It's easy to latch onto, and it can comfortably change your whole life. There's no law against having a good time if you do it quietly and legally, yet with certain enthusiasm.

You will have reached the epitome of joy when you can say to yourself as you prepare to go to some event, "I am going to have a pleasant time. There isn't *anything* that's going to spoil my pleasure. I have no responsibility except to enjoy myself. I am not in charge of a meeting. I don't have to make a speech. All I have to do is quietly sit

❖

back and enjoy myself." You do not have to become tense for any reason. Relax. You can condition yourself to have a positive time no matter what you do, and don't think that other people won't begin to sense this and be drawn to you. They will.

4
It's Not Impolite To Point If you Point In The Right Direction

It's a strange thing, but the public and your friends and acquaintances will go in the direction you point them.

If you have a pretty good opinion of yourself–if you honestly try to be interesting, kind, outgoing and understanding–then, if you try hard enough, *that* is the person they perceive.

We seek other human beings; we are naturally gregarious, and no man is an island, but we seek persons with whom we can relate, hoping that their brightness is a reflection of us.

I dare you to tell me that the sour, negative complainer appeals to you as a friend.

There's so much fun, so much humor in the world. It's free and it's all there for you to enjoy. If you're not quick to recognize it, cultivate and develop an awareness of how to have fun. It's amazing how much humor you will find in ordinary and also in unexpected places.

Not only is humor delightful, but it can change your life.

Laughter has a healing quality, and a sense of fun, of laughter, is so important.

Teach yourself to ferret out humor and enjoy it to its fullest.

Humor is often found in unusual places. Remember, there's no law against it, no matter where it is found. The only rule is: "Enjoy It!"

7

5
There's No Toilet Paper
Stuck To Your Shoe

Don't belittle yourself.

Why put yourself in second class when there's plenty of room in first class. If your mind can't preconceive it, then it can't happen—you must get the thought or the idea first.

You can't do anything without first telling your brain that this is what you want. Once you do that, you will be amazed at the speed with which the idea is absorbed and, in most cases, enacted.

When I was very young, the Saturday night dance date was the most important event of the week. One girl was very popular. Her dances were all taken far in advance and she was "broken in on" every few steps.

One evening during intermission, she went to the rest room. When she came out, there was about a foot-long strip of toilet paper stuck to the sole of her shoe. She walked back and forth across the dance floor visiting friends with the good old toilet paper trailing behind her like a bridal train.

I should have told her, but I was very young and at this time had very little character. Instead, I was happy.

When someone finally told her, she was so embarrassed that she sat out the rest of the dances, left early, and didn't show up for the next few Saturday nights.

Her humiliation knew no bounds, but eventually, of course, she got over it.

Now I Want to Tell You Something: *You* have no toilet paper stuck to the sole of your shoe!

Please don't look for excuses to put yourself down.

6
Sometimes It's All Right To Call Names

If you must speak to someone on the phone to place an order, to correct something, to make a complaint, to make reservations, please *always* get the name of the person to whom you are talking. If you have to call back or continue the project, it is immeasurably easier to talk to the same person, if possible, rather than having to start at the beginning and explain the whole situation over, perhaps several times. If you spoke to Carol the first time, ask to speak to Carol when you call back. She may not be available at the time, but then again she may be, and it certainly is worth a try.

In many instances, it is wise to tell her your name, too, so that if you call back, she can identify you with your particular request.

If it is necessary for you to speak to the manager or someone higher in charge, be sure to find out that person's name, and when you speak to him, address him by name. That destroys the anonymity; sometimes our actions are less attractive, unfortunately, when we are hiding behind the mask of anonymity.

If called by name, the person from whom you want an adjustment, a favor, a service, or some sort of attention will feel that you know him, in a business way if not personally, and will be inclined to put more effort and interest in trying to help you. Call him by name several times. It strengthens the relationship!

State your case softly, not in an angry tone. Don't be so wordy that you don't stop to listen to what he has to say. Be understanding but gently firm, and if you have a justifiable case, no matter how troublesome, I'm willing to guarantee you'll get results.

Try to get the names of everyone with whom you have dealings, whether he or she is the receptionist, the manager, the clerk with the special order, the delivery man, or the woman behind the dry cleaner's counter.

You'd be surprised how often this comes in handy, and you'll be surprised how often you'll remember the names.

It's a good lesson in remembering.

❖

7
Give Credit Where Credit Is Due – Not Overdue

A friend of mine and her husband owned a leased department in a large discount house. They signed a contract to obey the store rules, keep the store hours, meet a certain quota, prepare their ads and promotions, and so on. It was a difficult job, but their weekly figures told them their hard work was paying off.

The executives of the discount house had their offices on the third floor. Several times a day, they had to pass through my friend's department, which was on the first floor. Never once did any of the higher-ups say, "You are doing a fine job" or "Keep up the good work!" or "Your merchandising ideas are good." While my friend knew they were pulling their weight, and then some, they certainly would have appreciated some acknowledgment, some tiny word of assurance.

When her husband died, all of the executives, accountants, bookkeepers, and secretaries from the third floor came to his funeral. When she returned to the store two weeks later they each, individually, came to her and said, "He was such a great person. He was always so warm and pleasant and such a pleasure to do business with. He had such fine ideas."

My friend said to them, "Why are you telling *me* these things? Why didn't you tell him? It would have meant so much."

She decided then that never again would she refrain from complimenting or giving a pat on the back to someone who deserved it.

I have known this woman for years and she has truly made many people happier and given them a sense of security and a better feeling about themselves by just giving them a pat on the back when they needed it.

This is a double-edged sword. We all have a tendency to like people, or at least be more tolerant of them, if we think they like us. Perhaps we admire their taste. So please accept this little custom of appreciating your friends in a verbal way and compliment them when you think they deserve it. See what this alertness on your part to show admiration to them does for you.

You'll be surprised.

One of the good things about old age is that we don't have to go out looking for it. It comes to us, and it has its advantages.

A lot of the superficial things that seemed so important when we were younger are no longer important to us now as we realize their superfluity.

Old age gives us a sort of throne to sit on as we contemplate the desires and actions of those who haven't lived as long as we have. Believe it or not, it gives us an edge. We no longer think it's important to keep up with the Joneses. Let them keep up with us!

When we were younger, certain things were considered important if we were to be in keeping with our contemporaries. Who made those rules? At the time, we didn't dare question them.

Now that we're older and wiser, we wonder why we attached so much importance to such really unimportant trivia.

11
❖

8
Friendship, Friendship, Just A Perfect Blendship

All right. You are at home, comfortably doing something that you want to do. The telephone rings and it's someone on the line who would like to see you. He or she wants to be with you. You think, "I'd rather not be bothered. I really don't need anyone," so you say "No."

Maybe you don't need anyone, but maybe someone needs you.

Even loners need someone occasionally, and when they do, it's usually important to them.

Haven't you ever gotten involved in something that justly or unjustly put you in a bad light and was bruising your ego—maybe even crushing it? And didn't you wish wholeheartedly that someone would come to you and let you know that the problem was not wholly or even partly your fault, completely restoring your confidence in yourself as a useful and acceptable human being?

Well, when we accept such things, we must give them back, though not always to the same person. Don't always be willing to accept and never give anything in return.

The world is full of "givers and takers." The givers may expend more energy and some inconvenience, but the great inner glow of generosity and accomplishment that the giver experiences can't possibly be duplicated by the act of receiving.

9
Don't Be A Blabbermouth

If you tell everything you know—if you eagerly, constantly supply all the information—then you must talk too much. You should think carefully before you speak. If you do, it's difficult to become a compulsive talker.

Compulsive talkers are a pain. They never really listen to other people because they are so busy thinking of what they are going to say. They are on an ego trip, which is too bad, because nine-tenths of the things they say would be better left unsaid as their chatter has no consideration behind it.

Tactlessness is the murderer of charm. Being offensive doesn't win us any grace points.

Here's another mystery. When you keep knowledge—that is, important or gossipy knowledge—to yourself, in some mysterious way it multiplies like coat hangers in a dark closet.

You will find yourself learning much more by not being so verbose, and while you may not be conscious of it, you will accumulate more knowledge than you can imagine.

Don't give your friends too many instructions, and let's all try to be L.P.s—not Liver Pate, Lonesome Pines, or Library Paste, but a Lovable Person. That's all. Just a lovable person. It's easy when you know how.

13

❖

10
Bad Habits Shouldn't Become Good Friends

Remember that everyone is entitled to his or her own privacy. Don't ask leading questions about things that are none of your business. Don't you hate it when people do that to you? If people do this to you, don't answer them. Politely change the subject or give them a "turnoff" answer. Above all, don't lie. They don't deserve making a liar out of you.

If they feel that anyone has a right to ask a question, you should feel that anyone has a right not to answer it.

Also, don't be a buttinsky. If someone is speaking, wait until he's finished before saying what you have to say.

I had a friend who constantly burst into the middle of conversations right into the middle of sentences! She did it so promptly and so constantly that I couldn't take it any longer.

This is how I cured her. When she interrupted me, I immediately stopped talking, turned to her with a smile, and said, "I beg your pardon," as if I had been the one who interrupted her. Then I kept silent. After about five or six of these treatments, she has never again interrupted me.

Peace. It's wonderful!

11
Don't Be Guilty Of Accepting Guilt

Guilt is a negative emotion. You don't need it.

Don't have anything to do with it as guilt has never made anyone happy.

If you try to be this ideal person that we all love, there will never be a need for guilt, and if you practice the Golden Rule and take to heart the message of Polonius's speech in section 1, you will never truly have an occasion to feel guilty.

If you haven't done anything wrong, why feel guilty? Don't let others force this feeling on you. Look them right in the eye and realize that *they* are the ones who should feel guilt and not you. Why? Because trying to deliberately make someone feel guilty is an ornery, low-down trait. Consequently, you want no part of it.

Conversely, don't inflict feelings of guilt on anyone.

For example, if you find yourself snapping, "If you hadn't slammed the car door shut with my skirt sticking out of it, my dress wouldn't be ruined!" try to realize that you are in as good a position to see that your skirt is in as the door-slammer is. If the deed is done, your resentment isn't going to remove one speck of damage, which most likely can be corrected, so why not be lovable and say, "Oh, it's all right. It wasn't your fault. When the mud dries, I'm sure I can flick it right off. No problem."

The more things in your life that are "no problem," the happier your life will be. When you say, "No problem," really mean it. Don't just say it and then worry.

If acts are already accomplished and words or an attitude can't change the situation, then why waste time with negative emotions that cause bad feelings in you? You don't need it.

15

12
Making The Best Of A Bad Situation Is Making A Better You

Situation: Someone has found a new restaurant and enthusiastically takes you there for lunch. The chef must be having a bad day and his bitterness shows up in his food.

Thoughtless: "This spaghetti's dry. Not enough sauce, but it's so bad I wouldn't even want more sauce. The service has been terrible. There are spots on my silverware. They won't stay in business long."

Thoughtful: "The place is decorated in an attractive, colorful way. The menu sounds interesting and next time we'll order something different."

Situation: Someone takes you shopping and she buys a piece of furniture.

Thoughtless: "It's all right if you like the new stuff. My furniture's been in the family for years. Those marble-topped dressers were my great-great- grandmother's. They've got character. Not like this orange-crate contemporary stuff."

Thoughtful: "I think the piece you bought will look very well with your other things. If it's what you need, you were wise to buy it."

Even if it's not your preferred choice, learn to give a thing *good points* if it's *well done.* For instance, you may be a lover of tailored, contemporary furniture and settings and a hater of rosebud decorations and satin bows. If you should come upon a room furnished in Early American, with white organdy ruffles and crocheted antimacassars, don't close your mind by thinking "I hate this." With an unprejudiced viewpoint, look and see what the decorator had in mind. If it's done well, I don't care what it is, it should be acceptable.

You are limiting yourself when you say "I love this, I hate that, and that's all there is to it." That isn't all there is to it. The broader your viewpoint, the more faceted a person you are.

13
You Can't Applaud With One Hand

Behave in a loving way at the theater. We go to the theater to be amused. As an added bonus, we often learn things we didn't know; we experience emotions; we are affected by things to which we consciously or unconsciously relate. We sometimes laugh heartily, which is an excellent reason for doing anything. We may even see traits in a character that we recognize as our own or as those in a friend, and from this may come better understanding.

We are not always favorably impressed with what we see. Sometimes we don't like the subject of the play or sometimes we can't admire the actors or their acting, but when we consider the great amount of work it takes to present a play, there is always a reason to applaud.

Consider the labor put into the set. Consider the effort required to achieve the proper lighting and sound effects. Consider the many rehearsals, the special efforts to memorize lines, the stage directions, the blocking.

We may not like the plot of the play. If it seems to be going no-place but the actors are convincing, applaud the actors. If the actors are not the greatest, if they're untrue to the character or forget their lines or show a lack of interest, applaud the playwright.

I'm telling you *not* to sit on your hands. The dullest clods in the world are those people who go to the theater, who sit where they can be seen by the actors, and who, with a faraway look and folded hands, don't applaud. You can't clap with one hand.

If you live away from a major city, there is still good theater to be seen locally and regionally. Often the performers are not paid a salary; the love of acting seems to get into one's blood. Money is a small part of their reward, however. The reward is public acceptance, and that is why your applause is so important. If you don't show approval, it may be so discouraging that a young actor may not pursue a career. Now, you wouldn't want to nip a novice Meryl Streep or a Jessica Tandy in the bud, would you?

17

❖

There's so much good summer theater; it's so plentiful in the rural districts. As they say, "If a farmer has a barn full of grain, he gets mice. If he has a barn that's empty, he gets actors."

In theater you need three things: the play, the actor, and the audience. Perhaps most importantly, you also need the rapport between an audience and the actors.

Applaud with both hands, yell "Bravo" if you feel inspired to, and don't stay glued to your seat. Standing ovations say a lot.

14
Dare To Be Different!

A man had a valuable antique, a large grandfather's clock that needed to be repaired. No one wanted the responsibility of handling it, so he himself was carrying it up Fifth Avenue to the clockmaker's. A woman poked her friend and said, "Look at him. Why can't he get a wristwatch like everybody else?"

She thought he was being "different." Although most psychology books beg you to try to be "average," I don't want you to be average. I want you to be different, above average.

If you listen to the remarks average people make, they are often thoughtless or sometimes tactless cliches. They make these remarks by rote because they're the accepted—they think—answers to any given situation, but don't be like them. Be above average.

Be one who thinks before you speak. Either come up with a positive statement or, if it will add nothing pleasant to the situation, keep quiet.

19

15
Sneak In The Back Door - The Will To Change

Have the courage to change the things in your life that keep you from being a lovable, more perfect person.

You may not believe this, but your whole life can be perfected. All you have to do is *want* it to, and it needn't cost you a cent. No psychiatrist's fee, no hypnosis; no counseling; no self-help books; no therapy—just your own willpower and your desire to improve yourself and your own good mind. That's enough.

Who is that person who generates complaints, criticism, disapproval, or unhappiness? Could it be you? Who is that other smiling, attractive person with a warmth that exudes affection, love, a soft understanding, and a great sense of humor? Why, it's also you, or could be.

All it takes is strong determination and practice. Believe me, it's worth it. Your life can become a series of signs of affection, invitations, compliments, new friendships, and familial respect.

Think of the people you most enjoy being with and think of their qualities. Are they mean, complaining, griping, sour individuals with super egos and impatience? I'll bet not. If you have any of these qualities, lose them. Become the person everyone loves. You can be greeted with hugs. It's so easy.

Here's how: *Think* before you speak. Think before you say anything. Is your remark better left unsaid? Could it be offensive?

Could it create minor problems? Does it sound dictatorial or bossy? Does it have no point or add no humor? Then don't say it!

Here are some examples of things *not* to say. "You say you broke your hip? Oh, that's too bad. I know how you must suffer. Ann Marie broke her hip and she's having a terrible time. The pin has moved and she's in a bad way."

"Mary Catherine had a cold like yours last week and it's gone

20
❖

into pneumonia and she's in the hospital. You better be careful."

"Don't park there! Park here! This is so much easier. Take this place, even though it's farther away. You're being stubborn!"

"You say you're accustomed to going down Main Street but I always go down Market. Turn there and go down Market. I know you feel more comfortable going down Main Street, but you should go down Market. That's the way I go. It's better."

"You were a few minutes late when we picked you up to go to dinner. We can't go to the place we wanted to take you to because you have to get there early. If you had been on time, we could have made it. It's too late now."

"You're almost blind so watch your step here [said loudly]. Take my arm and hold the rail. Well, let them look. I have to talk loud because you can't hear either."

"You've redecorated your living room. Do you like this color? I liked the other way better."

"I like your new haircut. It's so much better than the way you looked before. That old haircut was awful!"

"Your new suit is pretty but everyone knows people with white hair should never wear brown."

In listening to what other people tell us, we are trying to get a true picture of what they really feel. If your tone isn't one that you would want to hear used by a good friend, then don't use it yourself. Manner, tone, and pitch of voice are just as important as words.

If there is an issue about which you disagree, instead of vehemently vetoing it by using a strong voice and an angry tone, causing a good bit of dissension, you could use a soft tone and admit to seeing the opposing viewpoint. In other words, you can always slip in the back door of an argument or complaint and win people over to your side.

Merchants are eager to keep customers; we are their livelihood. Most are willing to listen to a complaint if the knowledge could lead to better public relations. Of course, it depends on how you make the complaint. Don't start with a negative statement. Instead, sneak in the back door and start your conversation with a compliment.

Here's an example: "I have always had my car worked on in your service shop and I think you are excellent. You have the best,

❖

most courteous mechanics in town. That's why I was surprised when –." All of this delivered in a sweet, soft tone will get you the service you desire.

Give the impression that you have great empathy for the person or organization against whom you have the complaint. Don't make them feel that they are totally inferior fools and that you have suffered immeasurable damage at their hands. Let them feel that you understand their situation as well as yours.

In complaints with friends, always remember that if *nothing* can change a bad situation, it is foolhardy and distressing to dwell upon it or even mention it to the offending party. Some things can never be undone, just as spoken words can never be unspoken.

❖

16
Cultivate The Habit Of Happiness

You must have a good self-image. If you start to think of yourself as an ideal person, many positive things will begin to fall into place. When you practice good thoughts with positive thinking, that old law of attraction will start working on other people, who seem to sense a change long before you are aware of it yourself. Don't ask me how; I only know it's true because I have not only seen it happen, I have experienced it personally.

You have a right to feel at ease, and if you feel at peace with yourself, relaxed and unworried, you can block out every outside influence that would make you feel otherwise.

What are you worried about? Does your bosom form a shelf that catches the particles of food that should fall on your napkin or are you so flat-chested your blouses forget to bulge? Would your thighs be more becoming to a wrestler? Is your neck too long or too short? Are you too tall? Too short?

If you dwell on any of these things, you are being ridiculous. Richard Burton had always said that Elizabeth Taylor's legs were too short for her body. Robert Redford is not tall and Dudley Moore is definitely short, as is Al Pacino. Norma Shearer had casts in her eyes that made her look positively cross-eyed when photographed from certain angles. Did any of these imperfections keep these people from reaching the top? No, because they were smart enough not to let these issues rule their lives.

We don't have to feel self-conscious because we're not perfect. No one is. Everyone has little imperfections that we don't see, just as we have ones obvious to ourselves but not to others.

Dress carefully, see that your appearance is acceptable, then forget it. Go to the supermarket or to church or to a dinner, a play, a business meeting, or whatever. While you are dressing, remind yourself: This is going to be a pleasant thing. I'm going to have a good time because I feel happy on the inside. Nothing can spoil this unless I let it—and I don't intend to let it!

Cultivate the habit of happiness.

23

❖

17
Hints For Your Future Happiness

Life is like a mirror. It gives back to you the reflection of your own mental image.

Have a great image of yourself and live up to it.

Pessimism, greed, and jealousy are as destructive as bombs. They are the qualities that could keep you apart from success, peace, and friendships.

As you develop more confidence and self-assurance, you will have fewer feelings of envy and jealously. You can develop these good qualities to the point where no such negative feelings will ever bother you.

Laughter makes you feel good all over. Even though it's contagious, nobody ever died from it. It has no unpleasant side effects.

Learn to laugh. Seek out the fun in things. Once you become conscious of humor, you'll find the world is full of it, and it will start to crop up in unexpected places.

They say that music and love are two things that are internationally understood. *Love speaks all languages.* I'm sure you've heard of that. Laughter speaks all languages, too.

The value of a smile is priceless.

BOOK TWO *Mellow Maturity*

Zsa Zsa Gabor, when asked which of the Gabor women was the oldest, said, "She'll never admit it, but I believe it is Mama."

18
There's A Cure For A Bad Memory-
But I Can't Remember It

As we get older, there's a tendency toward forgetfulness. Well, it hits us all, and not all at the same age. Sometimes it even affects young people.

When we can't remember the things we want to, it's annoying and makes us feel uncomfortable, but it is universal—so don't let it get you down. If it didn't happen to most people, we would feel that it was a stigma, but it does happen to almost everyone at one time or another, so don't let it make you feel inferior.

They say the next best thing to having something is knowing where to find it. Even actors who are trained to remember sometimes forget.

William McNulty, one of Actors' Theatre of Louisville, Kentucky's most excellent, brilliant actors, was asked by a group if he ever blew his lines. "Of course. Every actor does at some time." When asked what he did, he said, "I simply stand and glare at the actor next to me as if he's the culprit, and the audience puts all the blame on him!"

There's the old gag about the actor who, when the phone rang, picked up the receiver, couldn't think of his lines and handed it to the next actor, saying, "Here. It's for you."

David Palmer of the University of Louisville Department of Dramatic Arts says that he was in a production of *Hedda Gabler* and at the end there was supposed to be a pistol shot offstage in the adjoining room. He was to rush in and then come back on stage and say, "My God! She has shot herself!" He waited for the pistol shot cue, which never came, so after an awkward, overlong silence, he dashed into the other room and found several stagehands and "Hedda" trying to shoot the pistol, which wouldn't work. As this was crucial to ending the play, he rushed back on stage, shouting, "My God! She's stabbed herself!" At which point the gun went off!

19
I Can Hear You!

Sometimes salespeople or waitresses or others, seeing that I am very elderly, will automatically assume that I am deaf and start shouting at me.

I'm not so hard of hearing that I ever miss out on a juicy bit of gossip.

When they start screaming at me, I'm always tempted to scream back twice as loudly or else to keep saying, "What did you say?" But this is having fun at the expense of someone who is trying to be helpful, isn't it? So I usually say, "I'm not deaf, but thank you."

If you do have a hard time hearing, there are good, inconspicuous hearing aids that will save wear and tear on the nerves of your family and friends.

Don't wave your arms around and don't have too many hand gestures when you speak. You've seen some people whose hands flail out in constant motion the second they start a sentence. Sometimes they actually look like they are swimming! This is not only most unattractive but it distracts you from paying attention to the words and detracts from the entire presentation. If you have to, sit on your hands or pretend you are sitting on them until you overcome this bad habit. It's one of the easier ones to break.

27

20
Don't Harp On Unpleasant Things –
Wait ' Til You Get To Heaven
To Be A Harpist

Don't complain. Don't nag. Be the person you most enjoy being with.

You couldn't convince me that you would enjoy being with a person who constantly complains about:

My children are so negligent.

My arthritis is getting so bad I can hardly move.

My son can't find time to take me to the grocery much less the bingo games.

The grandchildren call me only when they want something.

My daughter-in-law had a party and didn't invite me.

They never invite me. I wonder why?

Oh, the cataracts. I can hardly see.

Everyone's so wrapped up in their own pleasures they don't have time for me.

Is this a person anyone would enjoy being with?

Would you believe that this woman could be beloved and sought after? Would you believe that simply complaining is not curing any of her problems but is throwing her deeper into jeopardy and misery? Well, you better believe it.

What would cure this woman is positive thinking and a sense of humor, which in many cases is the opposite of an overdeveloped ego. She must learn that *worry is never the solution to anything!* Worry–just worry–has never in the world cured anything and has caused more grief and illness and bad luck than you could possibly imagine.

Part of living a good life is being respected, admired, sought after, and thought of as an attractive, worthwhile human being. You can be this person. You can often get cards, notes, or sweet messages.

You can get pleasant phone calls even from people you didn't think were interested in you. You can get compliments, invitations and gifts.

Aren't you getting these things? Well, why not?

I'll tell you why.

Every time you have a negative attitude, a complaint, or a squawk, you lessen your chances of being an ideal person by about 20 percent. Decide on a person whom you admire greatly and love to be with and study his or her characteristics.

No one is an authority on all subjects. Nobody knows everything. Don't take it upon yourself to always have the last word. Don't always be quick to express your opinion or make all the plans or decisions. The biggest bores are the people who feel they're the only ones capable of making decisions, laying out plans, and so on.

Backseat drive all through life. Sure, don't give the other fellow a chance to speak, much less to suggest a plan. You can always interrupt him. Every time he opens his mouth, butt in with your priceless words of wisdom. Abrupt interruptions are corruptions.

Stop to think before you speak, I beg you. At first, when you start to practice this, you will be conscious of it, but after a short while, it will become automatic. You will do it unconsciously and, oh, how great the rewards are. The tactless remarks, the thoughtless opinions, the offensive ideas are like the printing in the bottom of a baby's cereal bowl: "All gone!"

You're working toward that attractive, ideal person, and you've taken one *giant* step.

29

❖

21
The World's Most Important Location: The Right Place At The Right Time

One of the most important happenstances in our lives is being at the right place at the right time. If we're there, anything good can happen.

"I met this friendly little group going on this trip and they have invited me to go along. It's just what I need."

"That lovely person is looking for someone to lead a meeting or two. She asked if I would I please volunteer. I'm so interested."

"This fun group has picnics, square dances, antique hunts, and bingo. Will I join them? You bet!"

Most good things can't happen unless we're at the right place at the right time. We and the outside world are like a chef's salad and a favorite dressing. *We're no good unless we're mixed together.*

22
Beauty Is A Pigment Of The Imagination

This is for the women.

Now that you all are tactful, friendly, and beloved, let's look at your appearance and see if anything needs to be done to improve it.

Mother Nature was wise when she decided that light–very light–hair was more becoming to older faces than dark hair. There are many tones of gray and many tones of white. Never think that all white is the same color.

Now we don't have to constantly bleach our hair to be fair-haired, but if we are more comfortable with a tinge of color, there are rinses and dyes in light, ash-blond shades that will impart just a little warmer color to relieve the gray. Too golden a blond would appear brassy and unattractive, and even though you were a beautiful young brunette or titian-haired beauty, *please*, I beg you, do not try to emulate that color now. Black hair dye should never be used on anyone regardless of age. It is harsh-looking and will detract from, rather than add to, a pleasing appearance.

The ash-blond colors have been toned down–with a bit of gray coloring added to the blond. Some very pleasing colors have resulted. The drugstores have a large assortment of brands and colors. After an experiment or two, it will be easy to find a light, ashy color with which you feel comfortable and that may give you a tremendous lift. On the other hand, many women would hesitate to color their hair and, indeed, I find the various natural shades of gray and silver and white quite attractive.

So much for praising Mother Nature. Now there are some areas where I think she let us down and where we must give nature a little help.

While admitting that light hair is most becoming, alas, snow-white, milky skin does not make for a beautiful picture. At this writing, I'm eighty-seven, and I remember seeing corpses laid out in funeral

❖

homes before morticians practiced the art of makeup. Snow-white hair matching snow-white faces, in my mind, became closely associated with coffins.

As no one wants to look dead, there's an easy, harmless way to overcome this, which would make such an improvement in your appearance. It, too, is bound to give you a lift.

Use a color foundation a tone or two deeper than your natural skin color and see how much life this gives your face. These foundations are usually liquid and range in color from natural to deep suntan tones. Here again, you may have to experiment to reach exactly the color that does the most for you.

With this new flesh tone, you probably will want to use a tiny bit of rouge to give you an even, more "alive" look. Here again, you must use great caution. An obvious circle of rouge or a too warm reddening of the cheeks will make us look not only older but tasteless. Select a rouge that is only slightly more colorful than your foundation and place a tiny soupcon of it not only on your cheeks but also on your chin and forehead. Remember, just a tiny touch to give your face life but not an obviously artificial look. If your nose is large, tint it too. Contrary to making it more conspicuous, it will have the opposite effect. A white or very light feature extended out from the color-toned face will be more outstanding than if it were blended to become a part of the background.

If you don't believe that white is the brightest, most eye-catching color there is, plant a garden of brilliant yellows, orange, red, purple or what have you and you may think you have real brilliance. But add touches of pure white among the blossoms and see what happens! This is also good advice for trimming Christmas trees–no doubt about it. Add a few snow-white doves or angels or poinsettias and see your tree suddenly sparkle.

Black is supposed to be the worst color older people can wear. Black clothing, hats, and earrings are said to emphasize dark circles under the eyes and dark facial shadows or wrinkles. Black is a stable color, however, universally worn, and the advice I give you is to wear black if you wish but to make sure it's an attractive black, something chic, something smart. Perhaps that's why the basic black outfit that for years was considered ultrasmart and necessary in every well-dressed woman's wardrobe always included a string of pearls.

❖

If a garment is badly cut or doesn't fit well or looks shoddy to begin with, black will not give it dignity, as some people seem to think.

At present, there are literally thousands of shades of lipsticks. You have a limitless choice. Here, too, the dark colors are usually not the most attractive for you. I prefer the lighter, toned-down blue-reds rather than the orange-reds, but that is a matter of choice. A great way to get that glow of color in your cheeks is to use a small dab of lipstick and blend it into your skin. Beauticians say to always use upward motions so that you don't drag the muscles down. As you don't want a circle of rouge in the middle of your cheek, blend outward to the hairline.

If you want to carefully apply some eye shadow and tip your eyelashes with a bit of mascara, try it. If you don't feel comfortable with eye makeup, then don't use it. Your lashes may be full and dark enough not to need any makeup.

If you feel that cosmetics are not for you, by all means don't use them, but unless you have health reasons why don't you give them a try? They may add some fun and self-confidence to your life.

What we put on our bodies is as important as what we put on our faces. Colors are magical. You can do almost unbelievable things with color.

❖

For example, if a room has dark paneled walls, couches and chairs upholstered in dingy, faded colors, and a rug that is nondescript in pattern or color, someone who has a good sense of color can take over the room: the walls are now painted a beautiful background color; the couches and chairs are slipcovered or reupholstered in harmonious tones that complement the walls; the accessories are brilliant accent bits; and the rug has been changed to a beautiful solid color or a smart geometric-patterned floor covering. It is so beautiful that it doesn't seem like the same room. Well, you can do the same thing with your clothing as a decorator does with a room. You can be your own appearance-designer.

Certain colors seem to live a life of their own. Everyone does not have the same taste in colors, but there are certain ones that are considered so compellingly beautiful that they enhance whatever or whomever they adorn.

They say that if a person has been born blind, there is no way you can give him or her a conception of color, such as yellow is golden as the sun; rust and red are the autumn colors of sugar maples; or blue is the color of the sky and aqua the color of the ocean.

By the same token, you cannot give another person an absolutely accurate description of a color in words. You must have an actual sample. For instance, you may *think* the color "red" and in your mind you see a scarlet Santa Claus red, but when you say "red" to someone else, he may picture a maroon red. Without an actual concrete sample of the shade, it's almost impossible to impart color impressions precisely.

You might go into a paint store and say, "I want to paint my livingroom walls a soft blue, you know, a plain robin's egg blue to match the sofa. Please mix two gallons of the color for me." But unless you actually have a sample of the color you want, you may be creating a decorator's nightmare. You'd be amazed at how many variations of robin's egg blue there are.

There's the story of the woman who didn't pay her decorator's fee even after many bills and letters were sent to her. Finally, he wrote a letter saying, "Dear Mrs. A., If you don't send me a check by the tenth, I shall put a decorator's curse on you. May everything in your apartment turn brown."

Some of the most interesting apartments are monochromatic–everything the same color–but they must be skillfully done, with the one color just right, in order to be real works of art. If you want to try this, soft ecru, beige, off-white, blush pink, or dove gray may be colors to experiment with.

Some colors in clothing demand attention. A woman with light hair and blue eyes who is dressed in aqua or more vibrant turquoise can be a gorgeous sight. There are certain shades of coral or fuchsia that always bring compliments. There are so many beautiful, becoming, uplifting colors such as apricot, Nile green, all shades of blue, violet's many tones, creamy whites, beige, hot pinks, and geranium.

Avoid "dirty-mop gray" and other colors that can't possibly add to your charm. A light pearl gray and dove gray are beautiful, though. Light lemony yellows are a joy to behold and to wear, but there is a strong, deep "fried egg yellow," also known as a gold color but that should properly be called a peanut butter spread, that isn't attractive to anyone.

Too brilliant purples are too harsh to wear, though shades of violet–the many soft variations–are delightful and flattering. Lavender and hyacinth are also nice.

Navy blue for a completely tailored, crisp outfit–perhaps with a touch of snow white–is great. Deep, faded off shades of green are a no no. Later years have popularized wonderful, soft, muted shades of green, such as avocado, and lime, and the brighter shades of green in combination with other bright colors, such as royal blue or turquoise.

The good colors don't cost any more than the bad ones. Try them. Have fun.

Everything in the world has color. Even no color has some, and color can be important, as evidenced by the Italian peasant woman walking across the plaza with her very beautiful child. An artist dashed up to her and excitedly said, "Madam! I want to paint your son!" She said, "What color?"

❖

23
Be A Hobby Horse

It's time to pursue a hobby.

Perhaps you always thought that painting might be fun but you can't paint, so why try? Instead, take the attitude of the little boy who, when asked if he could play the violin, said, "I don't know. I never tried." Of course you can paint. The physical act is dipping a brush in color and applying it to paper, canvas, wood, fabric, or any background. The fun of it is the use of your imagination as you select a combination of colors, a design, or a feeling.

Have a model, if you like. Your model can be a vase of flowers, a bowl of fruit, a few dishes, or a half dozen eggs on a bright cloth. *Anything* can serve as a model. Even clear water has something to offer.

Gouache, a form of paste watercolor often used in primary school classes—we used to call them poster paints—can be mixed and blended the same as oils and acrylics to achieve beautiful colors. Acrylics are water-based and odorless; it's pleasant to use them and they're easily cleaned up after we splatter them about for a bit. Don't be afraid of oils. Some effects are more easily achieved with them than with any other medium.

If you don't want to invest in canvas, try inexpensive poster boards available in all art supply stores, most drug stores, and many groceries. There are many "how-to" books on all phases of painting, and there are usually art classes for adults in all vicinities. Try your YWCA or YMCA or some of your church or civic groups.

Perhaps you would rather start out on your own than join a class. There's no rule that says you must join a class, and you would be amazed at the number of artists who were self-taught and still achieved greatness.

Using photography as a model can be interesting, too.

You may prefer to play the piano, or the violin, the harp, the cello, or even the French horn. When you were younger, perhaps there was not the inclination, the money, the time, or the appropriate instructors, but now these things are all available—so why not take up any musical instrument you want and get others interested. The first thing you know, you'll have an all girls' band such as the Golden Charmers, the Tooting Tootsies, or the Arthritic Achievers or the Silver Haired Syncopators.

A group of elderly doctors formed a jazz band in my town. They perform at all the big social and civic functions, and they're having the time of their lives.

Wood carving, whittling, furniture refinishing, sculpturing—what an accomplishment to be able to do these things well. When people praise our handicraft, we may feel like taking a bow as an actor does at a standing ovation.

Don't forget tatting, crocheting, knitting, needlepoint, embroidery or quilting, and don't forget dancing. The most fun way to take exercise is by square dancing, folk dancing, ballroom dancing, and even dirty dancing, if that's your pleasure.

Many men never had the time to play golf. You have the time now, so do it. What about tennis, swimming, or croquet? Give them a try. These things can add to the pleasantness of life, if you enjoy them. And that's good. Isn't it?

If you have a heart condition, or any disability, please be sure to get your doctor's permission for these physically active hobbies.

24
Don't Invite Accidents – They May R.S.V.P.

I sit inside the glassed-entrance store in the shopping center and watch men and women leave the store and walk over to the area where their cars are parked. I'm surprised to see that nine times out of ten, they don't walk directly across the roadway to the other side. Instead, they walk diagonally, prolonging their time in the line of traffic.

Don't be a traffic lingerer. Large shopping mall parking lots are the areas most susceptible to accidents, so don't walk like an accident about to happen.

The kitchen, too, is an accident-prone area. When you have used the range or oven, always double-check to make sure the burners are all turned off. Get in the habit of checking twice; let it become second nature. You'll feel so much safer.

Be careful, too, that the loose sleeves of a robe or sweater don't drag over the burner, and always turn the handles of your stove-top cookware toward the back to avoid the possibility of catching your sleeve on the handle and scalding yourself with the contents.

Also, don't put things on the floor that aren't usually there. You just put it there, so of course you'll remember it's there, won't you? No. You won't. You're liable to take a bad fall, which is dangerous and unnecessary.

25
Safe Driving

When you are driving your car, if your passengers are chatting, telling stories, or otherwise demanding attention, it can be disruptive to you if you are having a driving problem, which might be watching for a certain address or trying to decide which street to turn into or struggling through heavy traffic or even battling bad weather.

Safe driving at times demands special, *super* concentration, and listening to or taking part in a conversation can be not only disruptive but also dangerous.

Ask you friends in a friendly way, to please be quiet until you can get out of the bind you're in, adding that you're interested in continuing the conversation once you've reached your destination safely.

No one will take offense. They will all understand the situation, and may even help you through the rough spots.

While you're driving, don't try to read a map or directions. Don't eat or drink. Don't put on makeup. Devote all your attention to the road.

According to Murphy's Law, when you think "I'll put on lipstick at the next red light," *all your lights* are going to be green.

Inadvertently you might run into some fun. As you pull up alongside someone who is pounding the dickens out of his steering wheel with a closed fist, swaying side to side (although you can't hear a sound because his windows are rolled up), you know he is hearing such rhythmic music on his radio, he can't sit still.

Remember, when getting into the car, sit on the seat first and then swing your legs in. If you can't swing both legs in at the same time, which is a bit more graceful, you can bring your legs into the car one at a time.

It is nerve-racking to have someone tailgate you when the driver behind you wants to go ten miles an hour faster than you're going, threatening to take you with him! If someone is tailgating you, slow down and give him every opportunity to pass you. Are you in the

❖

right lane? If he doesn't pass after you have given him the proper opportunity, then don't let him intimidate you. You needn't change your speed just for him.

I used to ride with a friend who occasionally would start driving very fast, and saying, "That fellow behind me is pushing me. He's right on my tail."

As long as you are driving correctly, the driver behind you can't intimidate you. If you are driving a bit slower, be sure you're in the right lane, so that those who want to drive faster may pass you.

If the driver of another car is courteous enough to slow down to enable you to change lanes or to make a turn or to ease any problem of yours, waving your hand or giving him a smile and a mouthed "thank you" is a nice thing to do. I usually smile and throw a kiss. It makes them feel appreciated and makes me feel noble for remembering to be courteous, in turn.

Don't you hate for someone parked next to your car to thrust open his door and slam it into the side of your car? Of course you do, so don't you do it either.

The time that most accidents occur is at dusk, when daylight just begins to get murky. Because you can still see the road, you feel no need to turn on your lights. Sometimes it's easier to see a lined roadway than it is to see a car in this particular light. Turn on your lights, not so that you can see but so that others can see you.

Considering the size per square yard, there are more accidents in the parking lots of the malls, at the movies, and at the shopping centers than any place else. There is less regulation as to how cars and pedestrians move, so drive slowly and be extra careful.

Remember, if everything is coming your way, you're in the wrong lane!

26
The Pack Rat (And The Editor!)

Me? A pack rat? I should say not! I hate unnecessary clutter. I like my life orderly, clean, and simple. However, I hate to need something and not have it. (Editor: *I certainly didn't want to encourage her to hang on to all that junk, but I hate to admit that when you throw something away, within two weeks you will have a pressing need for it.*) Having something and knowing where to find it are two different things. (Editor: *In her case, four different things. She has twice as much as anyone else.*) I'm not extravagant. I hate waste. I'm conservative. I don't like throwing away anything that I might have a use for some day. (Editor: *Like twenty years from now.*) But that's not being a pack rat. That's just common sense.

You may think those high stacks of old magazines should be discarded, but so many writers were paid for their brilliant ideas on all those subjects and there are so many good decorating ideas in them. (Editor: *Like "painting the outside of your claw" and "ball-footed bathtub and the long chain that flushes the toilet the same color to give the bathroom a decorator's look."*) Not that I plan to decorate any time soon.

There are so many good recipes and such wonderful things to bake if I had the equipment. (Editor: *For instance, a wood-burning kitchen stove.*) I'm almost tempted to start cooking again, which I haven't done in years. It's so easy to take guests to one of our good neighborhood restaurants. Look what it saves: no menu planning, no shopping for groceries, no polishing the silver, no ironing the linens and setting the table, no housecleaning, no kitchen cleanup afterward. (Editor: *When she's alone, she eats a sandwich in front of the refrigerator or the TV. If she has style or class, it doesn't show. What does show is the mayo that dribbles down the front of her robe.*) It's so comforting to know that I can have the know how in those magazines if I should ever need it.

Those stacks of newspapers next to the magazines? Papers must be recycled, and I intend to take them to a recycling place one

41
❖

of these days. (Editor: *If the fire department doesn't save her the trip.*) In the meantime, as my mother used to say, "They're not eating any bread and butter."

Now she was a saver, a real clutter-butt. It reached the point where we had to move things around to make space for the three of us to sit at the table to eat. (Editor: *With a little pushing and rearranging, four can even sit at* her *table.*)

The clothing designers purposely and radically change styles every year so that you will have to buy new things or look dated. They figure, who wants to look dated? Yet who wants to throw away all their clothes and start out new every year? They're bound to run out of new ideas and start repeating, and when they do, the perfectly good old clothes will come back in style. (Editor: *She has dresses old enough to vote.*)

I've always loved hats. Hats are something special, so I can't bear to get rid of them. They're so decorative. (Editor: *If they could breathe, they'd be collecting Social Security.*)

I thought I'd get rid of a lot of stuff by taking it to be sold at a consignment shop, so I took the stuff in. A lot of it. Oh, my. Those consignment shops have nice things to sell, and so reasonable. I stayed to look around. Couldn't help it. Everything was so nicely displayed and so reasonably priced. I picked up a few pretties to buy for myself as a special treat—you know, for my birthday and Christmas. (Editor: *And Easter and Thanksgiving and Saint Patrick's Day and....*) Before I knew it, I had bought more than I had brought in to sell. The lady was so nice to me. If my things don't sell in a certain time, I can have them all back. Isn't that wonderful?

My neighbor down the road is really a pack rat. He goes out and gathers up scraps of lumber, strips of moldings, cans, jars, bottles, screws, nails, metal, tinfoil, and street signs. Three times a "For Sale" sign fell out of his overpacked garage, and his wife nearly sold the house before he could stop her. He would have been willing to move but found it would take three extra van loads to move all the junk that he couldn't bear to part with. His wife eventually divorced him. He felt bad. He *liked* her but he *loved* the space she vacated.

Yard sales. Now, yard sales are something else. When people come and paw over your possessions and offer to buy something, you feel terrible, like you're selling your child. Somehow you just can't do it. But sometimes they bring things to swap or things you can

❖

buy from them. That's nice. It's easier to buy new things than to part with the old.

Then there was the man who hated the house he lived in and put it on the market. When he read the realtor's description of his house, he fell in love with it and decided it was exactly what he wanted. (Editor: *Nothing modernizes a house so completely as an ad offering it for sale.*)

Editor's note: *These pack rat people live dangerously. They are fire hazardous, accident prone, and burdened. It is hard to have a comfortable, carefree life with so many useless possessions.*

If they consider themselves collectors, they are mistaken. Serious collectors are discriminating. They look for quality, rarity, beauty, and/or uniqueness.

I beg all of these pack rats to unburden themselves. They will never know freedom as long as they are snowed under with possessions. Just getting rid of a bit of junk gives one an enlightened, easier feeling. Try it.

Please lessen your hours of labor and the danger of accidents. You'll be surprised how much better you'll feel. Being a pack rat is an addiction, and if you can get rid of it, it's a triumph.

Imagine that when you get rid of excessive possessions, you have taken off excessive weight.

Oh, boy!

43

❖

27
Into Each Life Some Rain Must Fall

We are not automatons. We are not heartless, mechanical machines. We are human beings with a mind and a heart. As a human being we are prone to emotions. Sadness is an emotion felt by everyone at various times, caused by a failure, loss of a friendship, a loss in a business, a loss of respect, loss of "face", a loss of a situation we thought we controlled. Sadness can also be caused by a loss of self-confidence, a loss of health, or a loss of some of our faculties. And the ultimate in sadness must be the death of a loved one. How can we cope with that, as sorrow is such a personal thing. There can't be general rules that apply to a bereaved one. The feeling is too individual and too intense.

Death is so final.

I have often thought how wonderful it would be, if when a person died, he or she could come back to life for just a short time so we could tell him or her all the things we didn't have an opportunity to say – things that were so meaningful – before death.

Death is a part of life, just as surely as birth is a part of life. It doesn't happen to just a few people. It happens to everyone.

You grieve over the loss of a loved one. That is not unnatural. It can be a sort of comfort to you. I would be the most stupid, heartless person in the world if I told you it was wrong to experience a period of grief over the loss of a loved one.

After a while, you will realize that there is a need for an adjustment. You will recognize that this person is not coming back. You will latch onto a symbol of faith or of hope. You will realize that you must go on with your life as the deceased would have wished you to. You can't bury yourself with the dead.

After the death of a loved one, many people go through a period of feeling guilty. Why is he gone and I'm still here? I was not with him at the very end when he needed me. I could have done more. I was not always easy to get along with. There were disagreements. Perhaps if I had done this or that, he would still be here. I never, often enough, told him how good he was or how much he meant to me. I never thanked him enough.

Well, I'll tell you, very few relationships are story-book perfect. It's the conflict and pull that make the good parts better. Don't blame yourself now for things that you may or may not have done.

If it is any comfort to you, most everyone goes through a guilt stage after someone's death. What's passed is past. There isn't any way you can change it. *But you can profit by it.*

In all your present or future relationships, be a little softer. Be more understanding. Be a gentler, happier person. If you wish, *dedicate* this new feeling of humanity and love to the beloved one you lost. The spirit of that person will be with you more strongly than ever, and you will begin to experience extra support.

Many religions have their own tenets about life after death; although, no one really knows for sure what happens. By all means, believe in the thing that is most comforting to you. But don't give anyone who thinks differently from you an argument. You are each entitled to feel the way that is most comforting.

I am so sorry; how can I express it?

It is when we verbalize too freely that we are liable to say the wrong thing.

Death is such a profoundly emotional situation.

It seems that there is nothing serious enough or important enough for us to say.

Try taking the griever's hands in both of yours and lightly press them. Look the person straight in the eyes and you won't have to say a word. You have expressed your sympathy silently. Or you may say "so sorry." That is all that's necessary.

If you are a close friend, you may offer to help send out the condolence cards. Or, if there are out-of-town guests, it would be considerate to take over a favorite casserole or dessert or offer to take them to a quiet place for lunch or dinner—whatever suits you and their lifestyle.

In some cases, just a trip to the grocery or some other necessary trip could be a big help.

The most important thing you can do at this time is just to be there. Just listen.

Later, don't forget the little friendly gestures, such as an engagement for lunch or a concert or to meet some new people. Although at first your proposals may be rejected, keep trying. After a while there is an acceptance that death is final.

Now hopefully comes the period of peace and readjustment.

He or she would have wanted you to continue your life in a productive, happy way.

Think often of the person you loved and know that the way you are living has his or her approval. Being kind, doing pleasant things for other people and yourself, having confidence in the good things you create and in your self, appreciating humor, laughter –these are not evil things to enjoy. These are fine, constructive things. You are not being thoughtless, and you are not committing a sin. You are being an intelligent, understanding human being which is one of the highest forms of life.

Please, I beg you, pick up the shreds and continue your life in a wholesome, *enjoyable* way. Please, don't allow deep grief and a situation in which all the grief and unhappiness in the world can't change. The situation is never going to change on its own. It can't. But you can change.

You always have a choice. You can sit back in a corner and mope and let life pass you by. Or you can be the wonderful person the departed would want you to be.

46

BOOK THREE   *Memories*

It's all right to live in the past,
but let's not be afraid of the present,
and let's look forward to the future.

Our memories may be old, but
our hopes must be young.

God gave us memory so that
we might have roses and birds in
December.

— Selma Jacob

28
Dr. Spock's in a State Of Shock

I came from a home that was not exactly broken but I'd say that it was badly bent.

When I was two years old, my father died, leaving a wife who was so in love with him that she vowed life would never have an opportunity to hurt her again. Though she was not an unattractive woman, she never, as long as she lived, took an interest in another man.

At my father's grave, his two parents made a vow to look out for me, and look out for me they did, in their own fashion!

I had two unconventional, ahead-of-their-times, think-for-themselves people to rear and educate me. These two could not have fit into a grandparent mold even with a lot of pushing and shoving. Their creed was "Do good if you must. Have fun, positively, as long as it isn't harmful to anyone, and the devil take the hindmost."

One Saturday, my mother called my grandmother and asked her to take care of me for a while that evening. "Sure. Bring her over," grandmother replied. Now it happened that my grandparents had a box reserved for every Saturday night at the Gayety, a burlesque theater on Jefferson Street close to Fourth, in Louisville, Kentucky. When the time came to depart for the theater, I heard some muttered remarks, such as, "She's so young. She won't understand. She'll probably fall asleep." Well, I loved it, and I did understand. I understood that if you want people to laugh, you've got to know how to tell a story. If you're dancing in a chorus line, you better know the routine or you'll make yourself ridiculous and spoil the show. As for the "bumps and grinds," any small child who has a Hula-Hoop does grinds that would make Gypsy Rose Lee look like Rebecca of Sunnybrook Farm. Indeed, I didn't give these things any more thought than that, and I learned something that is an important thing in my life now. I became completely fascinated by the theater, a fascination that keeps growing stronger and that has enriched my life immensely.

The family home at the time my father died was large, white, neoclassic brick with a Greek-columned square entrance facing a round grove of silver maples. To the right of the entrance was a large old lilac bush that housed a nest of beautiful but mean blue jays, and I was warned not to go near it. This place was called Greenberg's Station, and it seemed very far from town in those days. The house sat on about three hundred acres on which my grandfather raised wheat, oats, lespedeza, and racehorses. The surrounding farms all had lovely fruit orchards. It was the bane of my grandfather's existence that he was not able to establish a bountiful fruit orchard, try as he might.

My grandmother was a fabulous cook and set a wonderful table. She supervised the seasoning and the beginning of the preparation and then left it to Mattie, the cook, and Phoenie, the maid, to finish and serve the meal.

My grandfather was not always the most considerate man in the world in that he often brought friends from town to join us at dinner without notifying my grandmother. One day as my grandmother was riding to town on the interurban (a rural sort of trolley car) with a friend, the conductor overhead her complain of my grandfather's habit. From that day on, when my grandfather brought guests to dinner, the conductor gave an extra toot for each extra person who got off, and my grandmother would dash about saying, "Wasn't that three toots? Phoenie, hurry and set three extra places." It took my grandfather a long time to figure out how there were always just the right number of places at the table. A glass of wine was served with dinner and a liqueur with the coffee. My grandfather preferred a brandy, but that was about the extent of their indulgence. They were not heavy drinkers.

Scoggan Jones and one or two other neighbors went in for raising racehorses, but most of the adjoining farms were fruit orchards; when the Fegenbushes across the road would send Grandpa a basket of their finest apples, he would take a large bite out of the choicest one and promptly turn purple with envy and say, "This damned place isn't good for anything but a cemetery!" He made the remark often and we thought it was just a "Jakeism," but he said it so often he convinced himself. He sold the place which became Resthaven Memorial Park,

❖

a cemetery, and indeed the many souls resting under the mighty oak trees are in that peaceful spot because Grandpa Greenberg couldn't raise apples like the Fegenbushes.

The first numbers I ever saw were on a deck of poker cards. There was a once-a-week poker game at my grandparent's, and I was allowed to watch for a while, as long as I didn't stand behind someone and read out their hand just as the final betting was about to begin, as I once did. The first day I went to kindergarten, the teacher said, "Selma, can you count to five?" and I said, "Sure. Ace, deuce, trey, four, five." She shot me a startled look that made me feel she must have been one lousy poker player. Well, what did she expect? A royal flush?

I really learned arithmetic off the tote-board at Churchill Downs where the Kentucky Derby is run, and when the teacher expected me to give the answer to an arithmetic question, before I'd answer, I'd say, "What are the odds?"

When the races were in town, my grandfather seldom missed a day and my grandmother never. I would run through the house yelling, "Where's Grandma?" and Mattie would say "Hush, child. Don't disturb your grandma. She's locked in her sitting room studying her Bible."

The truth was, she was sitting at her desk surrounded by tout sheets and racing forms, trying to dope out the afternoon's entries. In those days, this was the main meaning of the word dope.

My grandfather never failed to admire a well-turned ankle. My grandmother, too, admired a well-turned ankle, only in her case, it had to belong to a horse.

As race time approached, my grandmother would slip into a tailored gray woolen suit and shoes with uppers made from the same material as the suit, a product of Laird-Schober. Over her natural dark auburn hair, she would pull a close-fitting toque of pheasant breasts. She never used any makeup other than a little face powder as makeup was a sign of "fast women." A friend of hers went to Paris and had her face enameled; thereafter her name was only whispered behind a discreet hand. My grandmother, though, thought that anything anyone did for self-improvement, such as a college course, a face-lift, or a loss of weight, was not only acceptable but commendable.

Grandmother never became emotional if her horse lost. If it won, as it trotted back from the finish line to the judge's stand, she would quietly stand and with all the dignity of the Pope in full regalia, she would salute the horse and say, barely audibly, of the jockey, "Good boy!"

My grandparents taught me that if you lose, you don't cry about it. If you learn something from the loss, it becomes an asset. Above all, high spirits and positive thinking are of prime importance. "Promise you will never let yourself get saddled with people with a warped personality, who feel that everything negative going on in their lives is of prime importance to you. Avoid compulsive talkers who pass right by the point and go on and on. They are strictly on an ego trip, and there's no room in their monologue for you. Never feel any animosity for someone who bests you in your particular field. To do so puts you in a position of envy or jealousy, and these are two of the nastiest, most destructive qualities a person can have. Above all, if without hurting anyone else you have an opportunity to put some fun into your life and you don't do it, you have cheated yourself and those around you."

As my grandmother said to her family, "When I told your father the Sunday night poker games and dinner parties were getting so large they were becoming cumbersome, I expected him to cut the guest list. I did not expect him to go out and buy the Galt House Hotel."

But buy the Galt House he did, the second one at First and Main where Belknaps was. That started a whole new ball game, but that's a tale for another time (see section 29). The hotel had a side entrance on First Street, and since there was no air- conditioning, every evening my grandfather and his cronies would have the large grillroom chairs carried out to the curb, and they would sit there and chew the fat and enjoy the cool breezes that obligingly rose up from the river a couple of blocks down the hill. As the evening wore on, the men would leave and my grandfather would continue to sit there until he fell asleep. When it got quite late, my grandmother would send for Josh, the sixty-five-year-old black "bellboy," to go down and tell Mr. Greenberg that it was time for him to come home. My grandmother would stand tapping her foot at the door, and every evening the same conversation took place. "Jake, you know you shouldn't be sleeping out there in the gutter by yourself. Someday you're going to wake up with your throat cut. Why do you do it?" And he would say, "Mary,

❖

it's so cool out there and calm and peaceful and quiet." My grandmother would shoot him a look and be still, but the next night the whole scene would be reenacted.

The Ohio River right there at the foot of First Street was the scene of all the baptism services for the black churches, and every Sunday I would go down to the river, get in the very first row, and sing the hymns louder than any of the members. Sometimes I'd drown them out! I was absolutely fascinated by the way the minister grasped the zealot by the back of the neck and drew him backward under the water, semisupporting him with his other hand. This was dramatic stuff, and I thought about it a great deal.

One day I said to my little cousin Louise, "Wanna take a walk with me?" She trustingly put her hand in mine and off we started down the hill to the river. We had just stepped into the water, and I had a firm grip on the back of her neck when I saw Anna, her nurse, come flying down the street screaming, "For God's sake, what are you doing? Bring that child back here!" By a fraction of a second, she kept Louise from becoming a Baptist.

My grandparents really believed that worry, complaining and negative thinking could lead to illness, unhappiness, and a loss of friends. They truly believed that misery was an unnecessary mental state not acceptable under any circumstances.

These two people had lost their two beloved only sons within six months. Their thoughts never changed.

So here I am—a product of these people who were so avant garde that time hasn't caught up with them yet.

And you know what?

It ain't bad.

29
The 15-Cent Soda Kid (A Sodaphile)

When they say, "Those were the good old days," do they mean everything was better then?

The Seelbach Hotel and I were born in the same year, 1905.

The first words I uttered were "six, five, three, two," spoken into a tall, black instrument that was called a telephone. That was the number of Grandpa's jewelry store, which was on Market Street, near Third, right next to a men's clothing store called Levy Brothers.

Across the street was my favorite shopping place, a confectionery known as Rudolph and Bauer's. They made all of their own candy and ice cream on the premises, and it was unofficially claimed, but generally accepted, as the most delectable parlor of self-indulgence in the neighborhood. Seventh Street and Green Street (renamed Liberty Street after World War I) were noted for other physical indulgences.

Rudolph and Bauer's made a chocolate soda addict of me at the age of three, and to this day, I have never found a cure for the addiction. At that time, someone had to boost me up. I needed help to get up on the tall stationary counter stool. Once up, I needed no help. From the time the fountain girl set that luscious, frothy, godlike nectar in front of me until I began making vulgar sounds through the straws, indicating that my ecstasy was at an end, I was transported to Nirvana.

Ice cream sodas were fifteen cents, after they had gone up a nickel, and there was no cashier, you laid your money on the marble counter, and it was eventually picked up by the fountain girl. One afternoon, my mother and I were absorbed in our sodas when a fire broke out in the back, in the candy kitchen. The manager came rushing from the kitchen, dashing through the store shouting, "Fire! There's a fire back here! Please leave now!" and everyone fled. My mother swept up her thirty cents from the counter. I grabbed my soda. I grabbed her soda, too, but I couldn't get down off the stool holding

53
❖

two sodas. I knew if I didn't abandon the sodas and leave immediately, I would have a horrible death and be burned to a crisp—but don't think I didn't deliberate and give it very serious consideration.

There were signs of the times. Business signs.

Every tobacconist worthy of the name had in front of his store, just to the right of the entrance, a wooden Indian, a life-size or larger reproduction of an American Indian in full native regalia. Tobacco was in its heyday, and some men owned pipe racks that held an assortment of pipes for each day of the week. Pipes ranged from corncob to calabash to briarwood to meerschaum. Cigarettes were prominent in the men's world, while the women were quietly and surreptitiously getting into them. Some of the more affluent male aficionados had special Cuban cigars rolled for them. Snuff was the delicate, affected comfort of the European elite, but here it was enjoyed by farmers, baseball players, and wrestlers, the simple people with no affectations.

Cubebs were cigarettes made from a substance different from tobacco. They were made from cubeb berries from India and were supposed to be slightly medicinal. It was considered daring for women and young boys to smoke them, so they did so in private. The boys smoked them behind the barn, where some of the most interesting things in a boy's life took place.

The rugged he-man rolled his own. That didn't mean then what rolling your own means now. They never dreamed of rolling dope in with the tobacco.

All barbershops were identified by a barbershop pole, a cylinder about a foot in diameter, printed in broad red-and-white stripes that circled around the pole in a spiral fashion. These were sometimes displayed at the curb in front of the store and later were wired to revolve. They were hypnotizing, dizzying things to watch.

The pawnshops all had three large brass balls, the middle one hung higher, suspended from a coat hanger-shaped holder.

The dentist had a two-and-a-half-foot bicuspid hung with a sign stating his name and office hours. The dentists at that time did not cap, do root canals, or implant teeth, but somehow they were adept enough to inflict just as much pain in filling and extracting. I had bad teeth and was a bad patient to match.

Most of the houses on Green (now Liberty Street) and Seventh streets had red lights in the windows or on the front porch. This was their district, and self-respecting ladies regarded these areas as a plague and under no circumstances would be seen there.

There were no side entrances marked "Ladies" in the red-light houses, as there were in every saloon. The side entrance marked "Ladies" was used by women who were "rushing the growler." They entered with a big tin bucket large enough to hold the amount of beer they needed to take home. This was the first "take-out" establishment. Even children could be sent to the corner saloon to go through the "Ladies" entrance for a bucket of suds. No IDs needed here.

No driver's license was needed to drive a car, evidently, because at thirteen I was driving my grandfather's seven-passenger Packard open touring car like a young female Barney Oldfield. I had been taught by an expert, and from the very beginning, I adored cars and was a careful, courteous, cautious, considerate driver.

This car had a windshield that could be opened horizontally to let in more breeze and a lot more bugs, neither of which were needed. There were isinglass curtains to snap into place to give protection from bad weather and yellow wooden spoke wheels to give class in any weather.

There were no expressways or superhighways, only country roads through arches formed by forest trees on each side of the road, laden with wild and rambler roses and honeysuckle vines. The view was of farmhouses set back on acred lots, horse farms, and rows of produce to feed people and livestock. If you drove long enough, you would come to a crossroad where there would be a general store, a grocery, and perhaps a small inn where you could get a drink and some food.

Expressways, while serving a great need, have caused us to lose the heartbeat of the people, their way of living, the feeling, and the architecture of the places we now drive through so rapidly.

All women had long hair rolled into a bun or into a chignon at the nape of their neck, a pompadour, or a coronet of braids. If some of the present hairdos had appeared then, people would have thought them outlandish and impossible, just as we would consider hairdos eighty years from now if we could see them.

Parasols or sunshades, as they were called, were an important part of a lady's wardrobe. At that time, the sun was not the glamour factor that it is now.

❖

It's true that ladies were admired for their delicate, fair skin, but I suspect that the parasols were not carried to protect their bodies so much as to protect their beautiful hats. Indeed, the hats, such as cartwheel leghorns with subtle dips and curves, turned unattractive females into femmes fatales.

These hats were beautifully trimmed. Soft pastel satin sashes would encircle the crown and, at the back, end in a large, drooping bow whose ends formed streamers that fell far off the edge of the brim.

Occasionally, a rose or other flowers would be added. All colors of lace, embroideries, ribbons and blossoms were used on these picture hats. Milliners know that the tulip in an arrangement needs no arranging, as it falls naturally into the most graceful position, as if it had a sense of good design all its own. Soft straw leghorns are like this. There was no way a leghorn could be unattractive. Would that we all had this quality.

For more tailored costumes, there were panamas or milans. Milans were of Italian straw, finer in weave yet a little firmer, and were great hats to sport a flat, tailored grosgrain bow and a face veil. Veiling was called "illusion," and create one it could. It was extremely flattering and could make plain women beautiful and beautiful women gorgeous. Later, Hollywood cameramen sometimes covered their lens with a veil when photographing women.

Winter hats were a different story. A buckram frame would be covered with crushed or stretched velvet or dark colored satin. The brim usually convoluted into upturned shapes that supported birds of paradise or egret feathers or pheasant breasts.

The only endangered species then were the ladies who wore the hats, but they always carried protection in the form of a ten-inch-long hatpin that was used as a weapon oftener than you would imagine. It could even be fatal. It beat using a pocketbook to whack the daylights out of an offending fellow, a situation that never fails to make me laugh. I love it. There's something so doggoned outrageously, indignantly virtuous about it.

The harbinger of spring was not a robin, it was a navy sailor straw hat trimmed in red cherries that seemed to be the uniform every woman wore to celebrate the end of winter.

The most stupid thing women ever did was to give up hats.

Every haberdashery-minded gentleman worth his salt owned a

straw boater, a panama, a homburg, a derby, and a top hat. Very few owned an English racing cap or a bicycle cap. "Casual" was not yet "in."

There have been many changes in food. In those days, when Mazzoni's rolled oysters were young, street vendors sold hot chestnuts, hot tamales, hot corn on the cob, and hot sweet potatoes. Every afternoon from two to five, a gentleman of Greek origin, laboriously pushing a large flat bedded cart, would park his wares in the street close to the curb at Third and Market. His sole product was fried custard. I began waiting for him at one o'clock. It was wonderful. What could a vintner buy that was half as precious as the stuff this Greek vendor sold?

In restaurants, every meat order was accompanied by mashed potatoes. Then the French revolutionized the restaurant potato by frying it in strips in deep fat. French fries became the order of the day! Their reign was long and seemed never-ending until the baked potato curtailed their popularity. Now seasoned rice and rice pilaf seem to have grabbed the reins.

Except for the push carts there was no "fast food." When people went out to eat, they dined leisurely and were served by waiters in black uniform suits.

The Old Vienna on Fourth Street, between Market and Main, was a favorite place to eat, and to this day, when I see bentwood chairs or hat racks, I think of it.

As you entered the huge double-leaded glass doors of the Old Vienna, to the right was a Machiavellian, evilly tempting display of the most sinfully delicious pastries on perfectly huge imported platters and great round plates, which later became rare collectors' items.

The French flans with perfect rows of glazed fruit, tortes, napoleons, chocolate-raspberry gateau, seven-layer cakes, eclairs— they were all there, demanding undivided attention because you craved them all. Selecting one was making the toughest decision of your life. After the manner of the Viennese coffeehouses, you told the lady in the immaculately starched white tucked blouse what your selection was—after three or four false starts—then you were seated at a table and your chosen pastry was served to you by your waiter, either as your dinner dessert or immediately with cafe au lait or coffee schlag (with whipped cream). Decaf was unheard of. If cholesterol was known at this time, it was like the village idiot—people ignored it.

Some of the world's finest food was served at the Old Vienna, and now, so many years after its demise, people still mourn its departure.

Mrs. Nichelson had a farm out on Bardstown Road at Fern Creek. She was a fabulous cook who lived in a two-storied, front-porched, pseudo-Greek revival farmhouse and who served family-style meals that you could die for. Country-fried chicken was a special treat then, and if Colonel Sanders and his seven secret herbs and spices could have tasted Mrs. Nichelson's, he would have stayed in the hotel business and bypassed chicken. The colonel was a fine, charitable man, and I am grateful to him for his chicken, but that's because I no longer have Mrs. Nichelson.

Bowls of every fresh vegetable grown on the farm were passed around, along with hot-buttered cloverleaf rolls, biscuits, homemade preserves, and dumplings. There was ice cream so rich it coated the roof of your mouth, always accompanied by a slice of white cake with thick caramel frosting.

The diners, on leaving, would hit the front porch, with the men all opening their leather belts a few notches and the women gasping in their tight corsets. Every once in a while you'd hear a prayer, "Please, dear Lord, if you don't let me burst this time, I promise I'll never do it again, and I'll come to church every Sunday." But after church next Sunday, everyone went back to Mrs. Nichelson's and did it all over again.

Teams of Clydesdales clattered brewery wagons over the rough cobblestone streets. The sides of the wagons were hung with extra-large casks of beer. There were frequent parades, and the shiny brass-trimmed wagons and the Clydesdales were always a feature. If you could get to a second-story front window on Market Street, that was the same as a box seat at the opera.

Open-air streetcars carried people to Senning's, Fontaine Ferry, and other parks on hot summer nights. These were minor excursions, but the ride itself was considered an adventure. Pleasures were simple then.

With no radio or television, the newspapers were our only source of news, so when things happened that were immediately important, the newspapers would speedily get out an "extra"–a special edition to be hawked on the streets right away. The newsboys would dash about selling the papers and shouting, "Wuxtra! Read all about it!"

Many things are better now, but some things, that are lost forever, were better then.

❖

30
Galt House

"When I told your father the Sunday night poker games and dinner parties were getting so large they were becoming cumbersome, I expected him to cut the guest list. I didn't expect him to go out and buy the Galt House Hotel."

Thus did Grandma Greenberg inform the family, in 1914 as I remember, of Grandpa's latest business venture. I was a small child at the time and knew my grandfather, Jacob Greenberg, had many business interests, but he couldn't have known much about hotel management—he had never rented a room or served a meal to anyone—but he was a man who took the bull by the horns and threw it over his shoulder, and it usually landed right where he wanted it.

The original Galt House derived its name from a Dr. Galt, on whose property it was built in 1834 at Second and Main. It became famous for its excellence and elegance, and being in the center of riverboat and railroad traffic between New Orleans and the North, it was the center of social and business activities. Every important person who visited Louisville at this time was a guest or was entertained here, and Charles Dickens wrote, "Never have I been more lavishly entertained and no place have I seen a more magnificent hotel with such beautiful appointments—not even in Paris."

On a snowy night in 1865, a subdued, anguished crowd watched the beloved landmark burn to the ground. Phoenixlike, the Galt House rose again, this time at First and Main, larger and even more elegant and more magnificent. In 1869, the world-famous architect Harry R. Whitestone completed the edifice, which he must have considered his masterpiece because for the first time he permitted a plaque bearing his name to be placed on one of his buildings. The Italian Renaissance design was inspired by Michelangelo's Roman Palazzo Farnese—the Galt House was almost an exact replica. The classically beautiful entrance had three massive arches supported by eight Corinthian columns that were hand chiseled by an Italian sculptor after the fashion of Callimachus. These graceful arches set a mood that pervaded the entire building.

Inside, the center of the frescoed ceiling of the huge black-and-white marble rotunda had a circular medallion showing Ulysses S. Grant and Robert E. Lee in full regalia shaking hands. Under the figures, in foot-high letters, were the words "United We Stand— Divided We Fall." I thought this meant if they broke the handclasp they'd be floor ornaments. President Grant visited Louisville and was escorted by a cordon of eight Confederate soldiers to the Galt House, where he was sumptuously entertained by the city's most important people.

To the left of the lobby, in a spacious, cool, less brightly lighted area, was the well-known Grill Room. It housed the famous bar but was a cafe only in that the food served was "free lunch." This free lunch was not the least of the hotel's attractions. It must have been the forerunner of the more stylish buffet, but believe me, the modern buffet is a weak sister by comparison. There were platters of several kinds of sausages, braunschweiger, liver loaf, souse, headcheese, pickled jowls, pickled pigs' feet, sliced cold beef, pork, ham, tongue, bologna, salami, hard-boiled eggs, pickled eggs, wheels of cheese, oysters—fried, rolled, or raw—crocks of kraut, mustard, dill pickles, hot pickles, coleslaw, spring onions, and all of the dark breads and some of the light. There was "Fish Every Friday." A wonderful, pungent, beery, sweet-and-sour odor permeated this whole section, which wooed and beckoned customers through the swinging shutter doors marked "Gentlemen Only."

At this stage of my life, my gender must have been neuter because neither this sign nor a similar one in the billiard room deterred me.

Ever notice how easy it is to rip the Kelly green baize on a pool table with the tip of a billiard cue? Grandpa noticed, too, and soon the billiard room was off-limits. I grudgingly understood that the Turkish bath and a few other sections were also off-limits.

The second floor of the Galt House had a grand ballroom with huge crystal chandeliers and hundreds of gold cotillion chairs. Before a dance, the white oak floor would be waxed and polished until it resembled a mirror. People didn't hop and stomp then, they glided. The bandstand would be set up for a full dance band; in those days, a "combo" was a ladies' corset cover and underdrawer garment. There were half a dozen parlors on this floor, each one furnished in fine European antiques. Flanking the entrances were huge bronze statues of helmeted Greek and Roman soldiers with swords and armor, and Zeus with a clock in his stomach. These men were angry, aggressive, and altogether too lifelike, making the second floor a fine place to bypass on dark nights.

Grandma and Grandpa were often invited to the balls and receptions, and while I was not invited, I usually made an appearance. As my grandparent's guest, I must have been the world's youngest and most frequent gate-crasher. I was usually quiet and mannerly and the elderly gentlemen waltzed with me.

On one occasion, I decided that dancing with a solar plexus instead of a partner with a face was pretty dull stuff, so caution threw me to the winds. I invited a schoolmate who was closer to my height–he was only three inches shorter than I–to come to a ball the following Saturday night.

That was a week of terrors for me. If he showed, how could I explain my bold, immoral conduct to my grandparents? If he didn't show, I would lose the will to live. I was about eight years old at the time, and I can truthfully say that never since then have I had the intense feeling of desperately wanting and just as desperately not wanting a thing to happen.

Freddy did not make the scene. I died of a broken heart. When Monday came, he explained that he had shaved and put on his other suit but his parents thought nine o'clock was too late for him to be leaving the house.

This second floor, which was supported by eight steel beams weighing 118,000 pounds, the largest units of steel placed in this section of the country, also housed a large banquet hall and about a dozen suites usually rented by the parents of the bride as dressing rooms for the bridal party.

An irate bridegroom, who was quite a dandy, was so displeased with the fit of his wedding suit that he shot the tailor in one of the rooms. The tailor wasn't exactly pleased either. There are so many tales about the Galt House, some of them must be true.

Madam Helena Modjeska, the actress, was a guest of the Galt House. Mr. Busath, the confectioner, created a masterpiece of a caramel and named it after her. This delectable candy has been nationally copied but is usually called a Majestic by people who don't understand its origin. Sarah Bernhardt, Lillie Langtry (known as the Jersey Lily), Julia Dean, Booth, and all the theatrical stars who played one of Louisville's two theaters–the McCauley's and the Jefferson–were guests of the Galt House. The hotel also had resident guests, among whom was Sally Ward Downs, a famous belle. Her beauty, charm, and exquisite costumes graced the hotel for twenty years. She usually wore large leghorn hats laden with lilacs or close-fitting toques sporting birds of paradise. Her shoes were always died to match her costume, and she was always accompanied by her maid. After Mrs. Ward's death, my grandmother became the owner of her tester (canopied) bed.

From the day the Galt House opened its doors at First and Main until the wreckers came, it enjoyed a reputation for fine cuisine. The first steward, Charles Claffey, brought his own French chef from the St. Charles in New Orleans, and the service and menus he gave the guests were unsurpassed. Every day during the season, guests were treated to venison, bear meat, grouse, wild turkey, pheasant, and so forth in the greatest variety. Occasionally, the chef would be asked to prepare broiled squab and a chilled bottle of champagne to be served in one of the bachelor suites; this was the origin of the "hot bird and a cold bottle."

Grand Duke Alexis of Russia visited the Galt House in 1872 while his father, Alexander II, was the Czar. He said that he had never seen anything in America or in Europe that equaled the excellence and the grandeur of his suite and the banquet in his honor. The menus were printed on white stain and the table centerpiece was a miniature (though not too miniature) replica of the Russian ship that brought him to America. Lines of waiters carrying trays high above their heads entered simultaneously from different doors, thus serving all the guests at as nearly the same time as possible. This last has been emulated by other hotels but I understand it originated here.

Savoyard, a Washington correspondent, wrote, "The New Galt House is a much finer building than the old one–there is no hotel to surpass it any place in the world–unfortunately it is too far uptown." Perhaps a bit aloof, but that might have been part of its charm.

By the time my grandfather took over the Galt House, old-time elegance was being ruthlessly booted out. Motorcars were nudging old Dobbin's backside. There was a Galt House bus that met all trains and my grandfather had a yellow, wood-spoke-wheeled Packard touring car with isinglass curtains that snapped into place in bad weather.

The beer wagons, drawn by teams of Percherons (rugged draft horses), still roared, rumbled, and clanked up the cobblestoned streets. Extra barrels hung from the sides of the wagons, and if the wagon was especially large and heavily loaded, sometimes there would be four or six horses. A brewery wagon in full bloom was an awesome thing. Often my grandmother would say, "Please be careful when you cross the street, Selma. There is no class in getting hit by a beer wagon."

Parades were the order of the day, and no parade was complete without the Percherons and beer wagons. The wagons would be painted bright colors, waxed, and polished. The horses wore harnesses trimmed in shining copper and nickel, and their plumes and head ornaments directed the beat of their movements in perfect staccato rhythm. No pale rose petal float this.

The American plan had changed to the European plan and there was not always a French chef in the kitchen, as once there had been, but the kitchen still was considered a good one and the hotel continued to enjoy a reputation for fine food. The menus were not as glorified as in the Galt's heyday, but they certainly were not as simplified as today's average menu. In addition to the usual seafood, steak, chops, and Maryland chicken, there was a full selection of European dishes.

The hot dishes arrived at the table on silver platters under silver domes; some were under glass. Café au lait was poured simultaneously from two special silver pots, one containing the hot milk and one the coffee. At this time, Caesar was an emperor instead of a salad and the waiter who brandished a flaming sword would have been ruled a hazard and ejected from the premises. Cherries Jubilee, crepes suzette, and plum pudding were served flambé but very quietly; no one thought of dousing the lights in their honor. There was a raw apple pie on the menu that I have never seen anyplace else, and I can't forget it. It was a brown-crusted pie filled with thin, crisp slices of almost raw apples, exquisitely spiced. How *did* they do it?

In the Galt House's waning days, even after the dining room was closed to the public, I still had my customary Sunday noon dinner here with my grandparents. Every Sunday morning, a lone cook came into the huge, vacant hotel kitchen and prepared our meal, which was served in Grandma's sitting room on an oblong, marble-topped library table that wasn't quite large enough. Dinner was always supplemented with superb rolls and pastries from the Vienna Restaurant, located on Fourth Street between Main and Market–and the food from the Vienna turned mortals into gods.

I am kind to little children and wipe away a tear for the last generation or two because they never knew the Vienna, never enjoyed that firm, close-textured, wonderfully flavored, braided white bread covered with poppy seeds or the crisp, airy croissants that left a dribble of butter on your chin. And the Vienna's dessert pastries! Large, round fresh fruit flans cut into slices and sold by the portion, with slices of peach or apple overlapping and arranged with the greatest precision, and the chocolate logs, each one with its own individual filling and frosting and as beautiful as a tax refund. How could we have permitted the loss of these wonderful things? Help stamp out chemical cream pies!

On July 31, 1919, the Galt House closed its doors. Activity had moved from the Ohio River and Main Street south on Fourth Street to Walnut and Broadway. Farewell, dining room–you were the best place of all- even better than the switchboard, the free lunch, or the elevator. (May the namesake of Grandpa's old hotel, the new Galt House, which opened in the summer of 1991, provide many generations with pleasant memories like mine.)

The day before the wrecking crew was to take over, a hundred of Louisville's most prominent citizens gathered for a sumptuous farewell luncheon in the famous Grill, the entrance of which was draped in mourning. They experienced not only lunch and nostalgia but also a great disappointment. The cornerstone, which was said to be filled with ancient bourbon, could not be found. The men stood with bowed heads as a band played "My Old Kentucky Home," the laborers dug feverishly, the sun stopped shining bright, and milady outwept herself–but no cornerstone appeared. To this day, if anyone knows what became of the Galt House cornerstone, it's a well-kept secret.

❖

When the building was to be demolished, the portico became the center of controversy. Preserved it must be, but everyone who had ever seen this magnificent entrance had different and voluble ideas as to where and how the columns should be used; as a memorial entrance to a park and as a public pavilion, were two suggestions. Each time a suggestion was turned down, the price offered for the pillars was turned down, too. Eventually, Belknap's used four of them in their new building.

Every guest room had a white marble fireplace and none were destroyed. I have read about and spoken to many people who claim to have an authentic Galt House fireplace, and I am sure they do. The Grill Room had a large-blocked, black-and-white marble floor, many stained-glass windows, dark, solid oak beams, carved moldings and frames, and a huge bar and back bar. The parlors contained many ornately gold-framed mirrors of ceiling height. Most of the washbasins were decorated with inlaid friezes of Greek or Roman figures or sprays of flowers. Before the building was razed, these treasures were all removed intact and were bought by individuals, antique dealers, decorators, and building contractors.

My grandmother loved beautiful things and through the years had become a collector of objets d'art. She accumulated so much that when she died there had to be an auction. In later years, I experienced many a nostalgic heartache when I'd ride up Market Street where the secondhand and antique shops were and see bits and pieces of the Galt House and Grandma Greenberg's prized possessions in the store windows and on the sidewalks. But who could have kept all these things? Where was the space?

Only in one's memory and heart.

31
The Day That Was Worse Than "Gloomy Sunday"

One of the ugliest things in the world is an oyster. The first person in the world who got up the courage to eat one did it because he thought he was committing suicide and sat quietly, waiting to be struck dead. When nothing happened, he felt that actually eating an oyster was too obscene a thing to talk about so he kept quiet.

It was centuries before anyone else had the courage or desperation to eat one, and he was a sailor who had missed breakfast and lunch before being shipwrecked on an island with a beautiful girl who gave him an incentive to live. As his hunger pangs were interfering with his other desires, in desperation he shucked open some oyster shells, but when he saw the shapeless, colorless masses, he said, "Aw naaw."

Then he looked at the girl and then back at the oysters, and he was so weak–both physically, from lack of food, and morally, from lack of morals–that he thought, "I must do something to survive–at least for an hour or so," but then he looked at the oysters again and said, "Aw naaw."

In the meantime, the girl's clothes, which were wet, were getting very cold on her body. Cold clothes feel as awful as an oyster looks, so she began taking off her dainties and hanging them on a tree. The sailor took another look at her and without another second's hesitation, swallowed six oysters.

The two were rescued off the island and the sailor spread the word that the world had been waiting for, that oysters had aphrodisiac qualities, which is entirely untrue. This fallacy persisted because it was generally felt that anyone who would swallow an oyster was certainly entitled to some kind of a bonus.

Later, more daring souls overcame their timidity and some actually relished raw oysters served in their shells with a hot sauce.

Then more venturesome cooks began torturing the little bivalves by wrapping them in strips of bacon and broiling them, stewing them in cream, scalloping, pan frying, and finally dressing them up la Rockefeller and Bienville.

In spite of these various ways of preparing it, the oyster did not reach its full potential until an ingenious cook at Mazzoni's Restaurant believed that if she could cover the little creatures so completely that you wouldn't see them until you were enamored of their unusual taste, maybe they would be accepted. She made a light but thick batter of crushed crackers and in double handfuls of this tasty coating embedded two or three oysters and deep fried them until they were covered by a brown flavorful crust. This was the birth of the rolled oyster–the one thing that lessens our sorrow at seeing summer end because you must eat oysters only during months containing an "r."

A strange thing about oysters is that no two taste alike. They all taste good, but once in a while you will hit one that is really superb. Some people get hooked on cocaine, heroin, or alcohol and some on rolled oysters. I was an early addict.

When I was a young girl, I had a maroon-colored Essex motorcar that looked like, and had all the charm of, a box on four wheels. It was the oyster of the automobile industry. The good part of this Essex, though, was how easily it knew its way to Mazzoni's bar at Third and Market.

There were always three or four girls with me, usually from cut classes at Louisville Girls' High School. We would draw straws to see who would have to go through the long beer-smelling saloon to the area at the very back to buy the oysters. They were put into a bag and wrapped in many sheets of newspaper to keep them warm. Generous handfuls of boat-shaped oyster crackers accompanied them. The oysters cost six for a quarter.

We would usually drive the Essex down past Fourth and Main to the Ohio River and park on the cobblestones at the edge of the water and watch the pigeons and water birds, eat the oysters, and talk about all the wonderful things that were going to happen to us.

One day, a friend of the family's witnessed our little escapade and promptly told my grandfather, who threatened to take the car away from me if I cut school and was seen in Mazzoni's bar again. I thought, "When he finds out how wonderful these rolled oysters are, he'll understand and forgive me." Unfortunately, he was already familiar with the oysters and *very* familiar with Mazzoni's bar.

About sixty years later, Mazzoni's gave way to progress—as they say—and moved into a residential area close to where I live. What a nice neighbor for me to have.

The inside of the new bar was bare and undecorated to the point of being spartan—no color scheme, no hanging ferns, no curtains, just the original bar from downtown, a cash register, some tables, and old-style wooden unmatched kitchen chairs. A cigarette machine and a small television were the only acknowledgments to the aforementioned progress.

You stand at the cash register end of the bar and give your order to the bartender, who puts the food on a tray, if you can't carry it without one, and you take it to the table of your choice. End of service.

You may have a bowl of chili always or bean soup sometimes. Oyster stew, fish sandwiches, and shrimp complete their menu—and I do mean complete. There's not even cole slaw, and nothing as pretentious as a salad or a vegetable ever got into this place. Wouldn't go with the decor. And a dessert of any kind would be ostentatious.

This is a place where you can eat and run and your hosts won't mind a bit.

One sunny autumn afternoon I bellied up to the bar. "Three rolled ones, please, and a cup of your surprisingly good coffee." The barman reached into the old blue granite washbasin where the oysters were kept and said, "Lady, you're getting the last three oysters we got. First time in a hundred years we run out of oysters!" Hmmmm . . .

I sat genuinely enjoying the oysters and watched people in the door smiling in anticipation, as people always do at the thought of a rolled one. Then the mood changed. "What! No oysters! Whaddya mean no oysters!" and "We waited all winter for a pretty day to drive fifty miles just for some oysters!" and "My God! They ain't got no oysters!"

Customers began crowding the bar, protesting, and if you think "the night they invented champagne" was something, you should have been there "the day Mazzoni's ran out of oysters."

Push came to shove and shove came to punch and two women —and three truck drivers—fainted.

❖

A hotheaded oyster addict picked up a chair and pitched it through the window. Somebody called the police. I picked two pieces of glass out of my oyster and calmly finished eating it. Kentucky has become famous for some fine things. We are blessed with a natural limestone over which flows the water that makes the best bourbon in the world. Our aged country hams and beaten biscuits are unbeatable. We originated the Hot Brown, Derby Pie, Benedictine, Bibb lettuce, and some pretty good horses–and Mazzoni's rolled oysters.

[This is nonfiction, but with a slight tip of the hat to imagi- nation.]

32
Crime At Gucci's

In Florida, Palm Beach's Worth Avenue is the South's Rodeo Drive. The most photographed people patronize these top-quality shops: Bonwit-Teller, with its violet bouquet-splashed awnings; the Findlay Gallery, with mirror and suede backgrounds more beautiful than the displayed paintings; the dozens of shops, each with its individual square or round scalloped and tasseled canopies.

Some of America's most prominent families have homes in Palm Beach, and it was not an unusual thing to see Rose Kennedy and her little dog waiting in Gattle's Linen Shop to be picked up by her chauffeur.

That she is a regular customer was proven by the fact that she called the salesladies by their first names; they in turn called the dog by his first name; they did not call Mrs. Kennedy by her first name.

Believe it, because it's true; there is a thrift shop nestled in among Saks, Correge's, and Magnin's. The humor of this shook me as much as finding a hot dog stand in Buckingham Palace. What thrifty little items would one find in a thrift shop on Worth Avenue?

Well, there are racks of still distinguished garments, such as Irish linen morning dresses, Italian slub silk two-piece suits, hand-woven woolen skirts from Scotland, and chiffon gowns, pleated, sequined, and embroidered. It was interesting to look at them and wonder to whom they had belonged and to which parties they had been worn. The beautiful quality and good lines of these clothes kept them from appearing outdated. The prices on the tickets were most reasonable. There was one big drawback. These belles of society never eat one bite between banquets. They're all size three!

The front of the shop displays butlers' trays, candlesticks, tea sets in sterling silver, Sevres vases, and bits of fine china–the prices on these things are not dimmed by time, and neither are they size three.

Perhaps the most interesting store is Gucci's–it has so very much prestige it has become a cult. You will enjoy a visit to Gucci's, especially if you like the letter "G." The letter "G" is woven into

71

❖

everything that is weavable and carved, hammered, or embroidered on everything else. I offended a Gucci associate (I'm sure they would not stoop to have a salesman–perish the thought–or a clerk) by asking him how much a certain tie was. All price tags were conspicuously absent, and the price seemed to be a well-kept secret. Stretching himself to his full height, and even standing on his toes a little, he looked down on me and said, "Our clients know that all of our ties are forty-nine dollars." Which immediately put me in the class of an Untouchable. The premise here is that of yacht brokers: "If you have to ask how much it is, you can't afford it."

Gucci's will give you a glass of wine or a cocktail to sip while you do your shopping. The merchandise is simply displayed and mostly unpriced. Well, elegance is its own statement. Preferred customers have a little solid gold key to an elevator that will carry them to the second floor, where the outstanding things are shown. Solid-gold cologne and liquor flasks, gold desk sets, bar accessories, jewelry, and household items (maybe *your* household), such as chinchilla bed covers, hand-carved ivory clothes hampers, jade figures, "skin" boots and briefcases, and so on.

Gucci's on Worth is divided into two separate sections. The first section is a store directly on the street. Behind it there is a very large open court; then the second section is at the back of the courtyard. We walked through the garden court into the rear store, and, after admiring the displays, we sat in a couple of chairs that had been placed at one side for the convenience of the clients. We had done much walking and it was pleasant to sit there and watch the customers for a few minutes.

A young man came in, undistinguished except for a brown paper grocery bag, presumably containing some few groceries. He walked along the showcases, taking an interest in several things, buying nothing. He spotted a low table with a display of several bottles of men's cologne. Putting the brown bag on the floor, he dropped to his haunches and picked up a large bottle to better see it.

"Look at that!" I said to my husband, "I'll bet . . .,"

"I know what you'll bet, but I'll bet you're mistaken."

By this time, the young man was carefully "casing" the store. I was more convinced.

"Don't you think we should alert someone? I hate to see people ripped off, even Gucci's!"

"I think you should sit very quietly where you are and ignore it."

While the young man swept the store with his eyes, I stared at him, trying to read his intentions. As his eyes came in my direction, I turned my head toward the yard. He began sweeping–I began staring–he looked at me–I looked at the yard. I began to feel as if we were at a tennis match.

When he opened the top of the bag a bit, I said, "Surely we're not going to let him get by with that. That's terrible..." My husband said, "There must be at least two people besides us in here who know what he's up to. You know a place like this must have security guards or store detectives. He's not going to get by with anything. Don't spoil the guards' chances of catching him. You just keep still."

I kept still.

In less time than it takes to break an egg, the cologne disappeared into the bag among the oranges and apples and our lad had hit the door and started walking through the courtyard. Faster than you could slip on ice, I was at the door, watching him. Halfway across the yard, he executed a little sailor's hornpipe, turned his head directly toward me, and with the most angelic, trusting smile, slowly gave me a most conspiratorial wink.

33
Sex Education

Kyung (pronounced "Young") is a very small, very beautiful nine-year-old Korean boy who takes Suzuki Method violin lessons on a quarter-sized violin Thursday afternoons at the Louisville School of Music. Often his mother cannot take him to his lessons, so I, his adopted-by-choice friendly grandmother, am willingly pressed into chauffeur service.

Kyung enters the music room, removes the quarter-sized violin from its case, holds it at his side, faces his teacher, and respectfully bows from the waist. The violin then takes its position under his quarter-sized chin, the bow is sawed back and forth, and a high-pitched, screechy "Twinkle, Twinkle Little Star" emerges sans any feeling or emotion whatsoever. That will come in due time.

He is an inquisitive, brilliant, and talkative child. The conversation, perhaps I should say monologue, starts the second he gets in the car. Usually it starts out with his personal Declaration of Independence: "If I was president, there wouldn't be any war or any trouble or any killing. If somebody wanted to start a war, I'd put in him jail. Everybody would be rich and happy and they could have anything they want. If they wanted a dog in the living room, they could have a dog in the living room. Everybody would be good and happy"—and on and on until you could in some way distract him or get him to bury the subject. The only trouble is, this very same dialogue keeps rising in the conversation—"If I was president, there wouldn't be any war or any trouble."

I know. I know.

One day he hopped in the car with an entirely different subject of conversation. His sister, Jeannie, is two years older than he, and she has sex education classes in school. Evidently, she shares her knowledge with Kyung, who is an apt pupil because here is a provocative subject that is new and fascinating. He talks in the same way as he plays the violin, without feeling or emotion—that, too, will come later.

I almost lost control of the car when this tiny child began explaining sex to me, using the correct terms in the most precise manner. He got along perfectly until he got to a certain stage, then "the woman's thing" gave him a little trouble. When necessary to refer to it, "the woman's thing" always came out as "the woman's thing" until finally I timidly volunteered a word. "Yeah, that."

A few days later, I became provoked at him for some little infraction and I said, "Oh, go on. All you do is go about telling everybody about sex." He replied, "I do not. I don't tell everybody about sex. Only the people I think ought to know about it!"

This child is nine. I was at least sixteen before I realized there was something more interesting in life than a box of candy.

I remember the guest on Johnny Carson's late-night show who said, "When I was ten years old, I asked my mother where babies came from and she said it was time we had a talk, and she told me a lot of the most amazing, most ridiculous, unbelievable junk I ever heard. And when I got to be sixteen, I found that everything she told me was true."

❖

34
I Can Get It For You Retail

Every day, promptly at noon, he dashed out to lunch.

The Brown Hotel Coffee Shop had a long counter with long-legged, low-backed stools. The rest of the rooms were filled with square and round tables and bentwood chairs.

The counter was ruled by two denizens, Marie and Lynn, dedicated to the needs of their "regulars" and specialists at serving those in a hurry to eat and get out.

A large round table was the noon meeting place for all the doctors, and there was also one for the lawyers.

The counter, with Marie and Lynn, belonged strictly to the jewelers and other merchants on that block of Fourth Street. The truth was, anyone who didn't "belong" didn't stand a chance of being served at the counter between 11:30 A.M. and 1:30 P.M., because every businessman on that block ate lunch there. It was turned into a daily social event with the same men showing up day after day, except Sundays and holidays, and the same two waitresses who knew their food preferences, flattered them, and cajoled, amused, advised, insulted, and admired them. Good humor and rapport were a daily item on the menu.

"Bring me some tomato juice and some strong coffee. I had a rough night."

"You sure don't look so good."

"And I'll have the baked sole."

"It don't look so good either. In fact, it looks worse than you do. Try the grilled pork tenderloin."

"Okay."

"And we have your favorite baby limas and asparagus vinaigrette."

One day, a customer came in and sat at a place at the counter that was always occupied at noon by one of the regulars. Marie, who felt responsible for her clientele, had to figure a way to recoup that seat. When she handed the man a menu, she said, "Oh dear, I'm so sorry you selected that seat. There's a terrible draft here."

"I don't feel it."

"Well, it's kind of an undercurrent–an *underhanded* undercurrent. Last three people who sat there had facial tics for weeks."

"I still don't feel it."

"I know. That's the bad part of it. You don't 'til it's too late."

Practically lifting him off the stool, she called to one of the waiters, "John, help this gentleman be more comfortable. Get him a nice little table for himself, a deuce on the Broadway side, in the window, where he can enjoy the–the–the–view–that's it! The view of the Broadway traffic!"

Sometimes lunch here was a musical comedy without the music.

The owners of the Kentucky movie theater took a small bit of their Fourth Street property next door and built a tiny gem of a store– so tiny that perhaps the only thing that could be merchandised there was gems.

The entrance door and the glass window together were about six feet wide. Indeed, that was the entire width of the ten-foot- long store. There was a narrow, specially built, four-inch-deep display case on the wall behind a specially built, eight-inch-deep floor case. No more than two clerks could serve the two customers who filled the store's capacity. Every inch of wall, and whatever else could be, was mirrored. Here selling was not the problem. Breathing space was.

Being so small, the store had no space for a rest room, so we had the privilege of the use of the rest rooms in the theater next door. Going to the rest room, we could glance in at the movie if it was a slow day businesswise, and if the movie looked interesting, we would sit in the movie house and watch it a while. When we began to feel guilty about goofing off from work, we would reluctantly leave and return to the store. Sometimes, after a couple of days, I would go back and try to catch the first part of the movie that I had previously seen the end of. Sometimes the beginning of this story was an entirely different one from the one I had seen, which often made more interesting, if more confusing, situations.

Because the selection of stock for a jewelry store is vast, it is impossible for most shops to carry everything available, so we played a game called "Stockroom Syndrome" or "Who's Got it?"

When a customer came in, for instance, and asked for a carat and a half emerald-cut engagement ring and we had a one-carat or a two-carat one, Hy would say, "I have just the size you're looking for. It's in the stockroom. Just a moment and I'll get it for you," as he dashed out the door to the "stockroom," which happened to be the ten other jewelry stores on the block.

The system was to stick your head in your competitor's door and, even if he was waiting on a customer, he'd look up and say, "Whatcha need?" You'd say, "Carat and a half, emerald cut, blue-white, platinum mounting!" He'd immediately search for the desired item. If he had it, he handed it over quickly then got back to his customer.

No one ever failed to help a competitor out. It was a gentlemen's agreement. I help you today. You help me tomorrow.

One day, a customer came in and said she had told Mr. Jacob that she would be in that afternoon to talk to him about having her rings remounted. I said, "He's back in our stockroom. Just a second, I'll get him." He had gone toward the rest rooms about an hour ago and I knew what happened. He had become interested in the movie. I entered the cinema during a dark scene and couldn't see the seats, much less Hy. I began quietly shouting, "Hy! Where are you?" and walking quickly up and down the aisle in such a state that some people got the impression there was a fire. Within two minutes the movie house emptied!

It took some time for the theater's owners to forgive me, but I'm happy to say our right to the use of the rest rooms was never revoked.

Installment buying was coming in strongly and it became our *bete noire*. How could we survive?

Because our space on Fourth Street was so limited, we rented a large office in the nearby Theater Building, which was a part of the Loew's chain. It provided space for our expert watch repairman and our jewelry designer, but there wasn't room for the files and equipment necessary for an installment operation. This was a cause of great concern for us. We both liked the jewelry business. We felt comfortable in it. We were sincere and had a good following, but if we couldn't meet the public's demand for installment credit, we were doomed and we knew it. What to do?

This was an uncomfortable period in our lives until, one day, Hy came back from lunch and said, "I ran into Jerry Gershwin in the coffee shop, and he told me he's about to open Louisville's first discount house. He offered me the jewelry department. All the other departments will be owned and managed by him, but he's not set up for jewelry, nor is he knowledgeable about it. We would lease the space and manage it just as we are doing here in our present business. We would keep our own watch and jewelry repair people." It was a way out. An answer to our prayers. We accepted it.

Life in a discount house was difficult. The hours were long, long. The regimen was strict. The stock work was interminable. The suggestions from the executives were stern and constant. Easy, it was not. Yet we both felt grateful because if we had not made this change, we would not have survived. Because we felt gratitude, we put forth a special effort to please the customers and to give good service. The only complaints we got were when watch repair work was not completed on time, which seems to be par for the watch repair course.

We felt that we must be pleasing our superiors because they certainly would not have let us continue if we were not satisfactory, yet they never complimented us, they never showed any sign of being pleased with what we were doing.

Hy and I had no living relatives and no children. He was my entire life, and the business was my only other chief interest.

My life seemed to come to an end the day Hy unexpectedly died of a heart attack after two days in the hospital. There was nothing left for me. I knew the company would want our space immediately, as it was the A1 spot in the store. It had to be reassigned at once; I knew that.

When I called Jerry and told him that Hy had died, he asked me to come in and talk to him at three o'clock the day after the funeral. I knew why he asked to meet me. It isn't easy to tell a person in my situation to vacate the premises, yet I knew he had to do it. I prayed constantly that they would give me reasonable time to dispose of the large stock, the fixtures, and the equipment, though I doubted that they could spare as much time as it would reasonably take.

I arrived promptly at three and quietly sat, my insides quivering so that I thought it must be visible to everyone. I had lost Hy. I was nothing–a lost soul, a zombie. I had lost everything. I knew I had to give up the business. Well, all things come to an end, and this was the end of my life, too.

Never, ever will I forget the lump in my throat and the gasp– like the gasp of new life when a child is born–when I heard Jerry Gershwin say, "We would be pleased to have you continue your husband's business."

35
Kudzu Imagine A Thing Like That

Sure the Japanese are doing good things for us. They're making us cheap cars and better lenses, and they're teaching us their superior method of assembly-line industry. They're even sending us an imitation crabmeat much better than the real thing.

You know why they're doing all this? Kudzu. That's the answer. They have a worse guilt complex about sending us kudzu than we have about sending them the Hiroshima bomb.

Kudzu is a vicious, almost carnivorous plant that was sent to the United States in 1930 to be used as a ground cover in Georgia, where it seemed nothing was powerful enough to stop the erosion of the bright-red soil. When the soil realized the shame of its propagating such an evil, it shrank in revulsion until Georgia is now half the size it used to be.

When my husband and I first saw kudzu, we had just finished building our hillside home with five levels of garden in the back. We made good use of pachysandra, periwinkle, vinca minor, and ivy, but the ground to be covered seemed endless. When there were strong rains and the rivulets of water and good topsoil streamed down to the very foot of the hill, we felt defeated. A couple who were friends of ours had been given a rather rare wisteria tree with heavy blossoms and branches and a very weak, slender trunk. They were warned that because of the delicate thin trunk, it was difficult to grow these trees to maturity and that in a wind or rainstorm, it should be protected. After that, on most rainy or windy nights, if you drove past their house, you could see the two of them in rain hats and overcoats—one on either side of the tree holding onto the trunk. It's harder to hold onto two hundred feet of sliding mud.

Well, as I was saying, we were driving through Georgia and I spotted this large bright-green, three-pointed leaf that obviously was a great ground cover and was spreading out in a most graceful way. How beautiful, how *strong* it looked. What a perfect answer to erosion.

❖

I said, "Anything that would grow in this red clay would grow in cement. If we could take a tiny start of this stuff, it would be the answer to our problem." My husband said, "It would also be against the law."

I said, "Of course it would, we couldn't think of it, and we haven't a thing to dig it with. Could you stop at the next hardware store?"

Well, to shorten a long story, we stopped at three hardware stores, each time buying larger, stronger tools because this plant not only had a resistance you wouldn't believe–it fought back! It first knocked off your glasses, then poked you in the eye. It caused you to backslide down a steep, muddy hill on your backside. The roots grabbed your ankles and caused you to emulate the man on the flying trapeze–your hands were bloodied and muddied and your clothing didn't look exactly pristine.

My husband, who had the patience and character of a saint (but not the vocabulary), was the first to say, "The hell with it." I was relieved to second his opinion and stopped trying to get a piece of this root that was like an oak tree. We didn't realize until later how wise we were to give up. Whoever said, "If at first you don't succeed" never tried to dig a kudzu root.

Well, the next time we drove through Georgia, kudzu had taken over the whole countryside. It had not only climbed telephone poles and tree trunks, it had completely covered whole trees! A car was stalled near this stuff for a couple of days and when the tow truck came to get it, they had to get fire axes and chop the car out. Some small barns were completely covered and people hesitated to stop and chat too long because this treacherous menace would grow in their direction faster than was feasible.

Unfortunately, this stuff is spreading to other states, and while we sure didn't bring it here, it has been reported to be flourishing in Oldham County. We have some friends in Oldham County who had a darling grandpa–Grandpa Higgins. There was a plumbing problem in the farmhouse, so Grandpa Higgins took a copy of *Playboy* and headed for the outhouse. Unfortunately, he stayed there a little too long. *Playboy* was too interesting.

They never did get him out.

Kudzu imagine a thing like that?

AFTERWORD

Goethe said (not to me), "If I love you, what business is that of yours?"

What a wonderful thing to have said. I'm willing to give you something and expect nothing in return. And how nice to admire or like or love many persons and not really insist that they return the emotion. Give them the freedom to go their own ways and give me the freedom to feel as I please. By not grasping too closely, we often hold the tightest.

Monna Fenley, a dear friend, wrote a little poem that expresses this so well:

Perversity
If it were of necessity
That I am true to you
The yoke would be unbearable,
My love would all undo.

But now that you have left me,
Nor care where I may be,
No earthly power holds me so fast
As knowing I am free.

Well, perhaps not the happiest conclusion, but it certainly gets the idea across.

Then, on the other side, Monna says:

A Gesture

For all those joys
Of which I take small sips
I sometimes sigh;
But I, someday, will raise it to my lips–
This brimming cup
From which my pleasure drips–
And drink it dry.

I am eighty-seven. Monna is about my age. Do you like the things she writes? Try your hand at it. It can be fun. If you don't want to go for rhymes, you can write modern, free-form poetry with no rhyming words necessarily. Simply write down your thoughts or feelings with a rhythmic flow of sound–cadence–it's practically prose and not difficult once you get the hang of it.

If you've ever felt that you were a real loser, and who hasn't at one time or another, perhaps you'll read these lyrics I wrote because I thought Cole Porter and Ira Gershwin were having all the fun:

Photo Finish

I'm running third in a three-horse race close behind
The horse that's before me–
I feel like the thing that's in front of my face
Oh, Fate, how you must adore me!
Chorus:
I get there first; the rest come late
I get there late; the rest don't wait
If I do, I never should have done it
If I don't, I'm sure I could have won it.
I greet a friend–I mean to say "HI!"
and accidentally spit in his eye.
I break my neck and everyone howls
When I'm with that special someone my stomach growls
But I'm running third in a three-horse race
In there pitchin' with a grin.
For Fate's a perverse thing–if she should reverse things
What do you know? I might win!

Winter is a cold, harsh, biting, unfriendly (except for ski-lovers) season. Spring is a season of renewed hope, rebirth, another chance, an awakening. Summer is the culmination of Springtime–the fruition of hopes and dreams–the growth of nature – the flowers, the fruits, the blossoming of all good and beautiful things.

If you have honestly practiced the concepts of this book, and feel that you have a better viewpoint and are a better you, then rejoice with this wonderful quotation from Camus:

"In the midst of winter, I finally learned that there was in me an invincible summer."

There is an invincible summer in you. Recognize it! Let it out!

Flare its butterfly-like wings to the sunlight.

Unfurl its banners in the breeze.

The warmth and radiance is there.

It is you!

You are an invincible summer!

Bravo!

ABOUT THE
AUTHOR

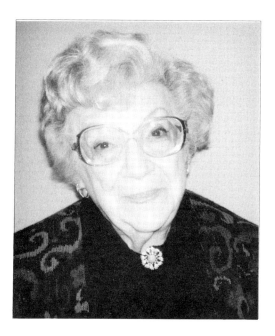

Octogenarian Selma Jacob, a life-long resident of Louisville, Kentucky, is the organizer of "Writers & Readers," a creative writing group, and a devotee of the theatre who holds weekly drama study groups with University of Louisville students in her home. Her love of the English language and dramatic arts was instilled at an early age: "None of us were actors," she says of her family, "but we were the best audience an actor ever had!"

Born in Louisville in 1905, Selma was married for more than 50 years to Hyman Jacob, and took over their jewelry business after his death, not retiring until 1984. She now devotes more time to her creative endeavors, which include theatre and writing. A six-time produced playright, this is Selma's first book.

Her inspiration for *Once You're Over The Hill...*, which she calls a "Renaissance book for older people" (and indeed everyone), came from a desire to help others "shed the bonds of misery and put on the cloak of happiness" and, she says, "the fact that my lawyer told me, 'You can say anything you feel like saying!' "